CANDIDA ALBICANS
Could Yeast be Your Problem?

Shows how the proliferation of the yeast *Candida* in your body has been found to be the root of illness where no obvious cause is evident.

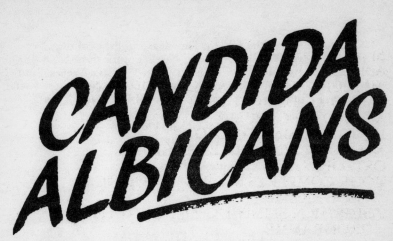

CANDIDA ALBICANS

Could Yeast be Your Problem?

by

LEON CHAITOW
N.D., D.O., M.B.N.O.A.

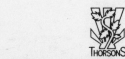

THORSONS PUBLISHING GROUP
Wellingborough * New York

Published in the UK by Thorsons Publishers Ltd.,
Denington Estate, Wellingborough, Northamptonshire NN8 2RQ,
and in the USA by Thorsons Publishers Inc., 377 Park Avenue South,
New York, NY 10016. Thorsons Publishers Inc. are distributed to the
trade by Inner Traditions International Ltd., New York.

First published June 1985
Second Impression August 1985
Third Impression November 1985
Fourth Impression March 1986

British Library Cataloguing in Publication Data

Chaitow, Leon
    Candida albicans: could yeast be your problem?
    1. Candida
    I. Title
    616'.015   QR201.06

    ISBN 0-7225-1144-2

Printed and bound in Great Britain

ACKNOWLEDGEMENTS

The pioneering research of Dr C. Orion Truss in the uncovering of Candida's involvement in a wide range of diseases and conditions deserves recognition. I would respectfully dedicate this book to him. Others who have made major contributions to this knowledge, and to whom I owe a debt, include Dr William G. Crook, and Dr Jeffrey Bland. I have quoted from all three of these respected scientists, and thank them on behalf of all those who will benefit from their original work. The books of Dr Truss and Dr Crook (*The Missing Diagnosis* and *The Yeast Connnection*, respectively) are worthy of study by anyone who wishes to have a deeper knowledge of this subject.

CONTENTS

1.

CANDIDA YEAST AND COMMON HEALTH PROBLEMS

In the very recent past it has become clear that a great many common health problems, both physical and mental in expression, might have a common cause – namely, the spread in the body of a yeast that lives in each and every one of us. Its name is *Candida albicans*, and we will call it Candida for short.

Because it is present in all people from about the age of six months onwards, Candida tends to become neglected in the eyes of doctors seeking the causes of particular diseases or conditions. Since it is in everyone, it seems that Candida cannot be causing particular symptoms in only some. This reasoning has prevented attention being given to Candida, except in rare conditions in which it proliferates to such an extent as to become life-threatening. This, interestingly enough, often happens in people whose defence mechanism (immune system) has become weakened by disease or drugs (in therapy or in abuse). This gives a clue as to why a great many people may indeed be suffering from a less pronounced spread of Candida, which, whilst not sufficient to endanger life, is certainly enough to produce a wide array of debilitating symptoms. These include: depression; anxiety; unnatural

irritability; digestive symptoms such as diarrhoea, constipation, bloating and heartburn; tiredness and a sense of
hopelessness; allergies; acne; migraine; cystitis; vaginitis;
thrush; menstrual problems and pre-menstrual tension.

The key to understanding the way in which this vast
array of symptoms could possibly result from the effects
of a yeast that lives in all of us, lies in an appreciation of
those factors which can encourage a spread of yeast. In
most people there is an uneasy truce between their body
and the yeast that lives inside it. Over many thousands of
years an equilibrium has been struck. The yeast can live,
and thrive, and present no problems to its host, the body,
as long as it confines itself to specific sites. Should it go
beyond these sites, the defence capability of the body, as
represented by its immune system in general and its white
blood cells in particular, attacks and destroys the yeast.
There are also actual physical barriers, such as the
mucous lining of the digestive tract, which prevents
intrusion through it by yeast or any other undesirable
elements. All mucous membranes contain further pro-
tective substances which can destroy invading particles of
yeast. We will consider these defences later, in our search
for an understanding of this problem.

At this stage we should simply have an appreciation of
the efficient defence capability, on the part of the body,
which deals with toxins, bacteria and yeast, should any of
them intrude upon areas in which they present a danger
to the body. The problem arises when, because of one of a
variety of causes, the defence capability becomes deficient
or weakens. Should this happen, the controls which keep
Candida in check would be removed, and it would be able
to spread to other areas normally out of bounds. If at the
same time the foods the yeast thrives on happen to be in
plentiful supply, we have the recipe for an explosion of
Candida activity. This is precisely the combination of
factors that has been identified as having become wide-

spread in Western society over the past twenty-five to
thirty years.

We will look at the dietary aspect in detail, and also at
those changes in medical care which have, inadvertently,
allowed Candida's new-found freedom from adequate
surveillance.

The introduction of broad-spectrum antibiotics, the
use of the contraceptive pill, and the widespread use of
steroids, have all played their part in Candida's growth. In
addition the increase in the use of sugar and sugar-rich
foods has provided the yeast with just the sustenance it
loves. This is the unfortunate combination of factors that
is the root cause of the problem for many people.

A careful look at the nature of the enemy is necessary,
together with consideration of those factors and circumstances which allow it to proliferate, and what the
consequences of such a proliferation might be. We will
then be in a position to consider methods of controlling
Candida. Fortunately this is the brighter side of the sorry
mess. For it seems unlikely that the causative elements of
the picture are going to be removed from the population
at large, and so the fact that control is possible, in the
majority of cases, is a blessing indeed.

It should be clearly understood that it is not being
suggested that in all cases the conditions listed above are
the result of Candida infection. It is certainly true that all
of these *might* be such a result, but equally there can be
other causes. It is the view of those practitioners now
aware of the possibility of Candida's involvement in
common disease problems of this sort that when a
combination of such symptoms appears in a person, with
no other obvious causes apparent, then Candida should
be the prime suspect. Unlike most infection and infest-
ations, it is not really possible to test for the presence of
Candida to prove or disprove such an assumption. This is
because, as has already been stated, Candida is present to

some extent in all of us. This would make looking for it as pointless as looking for mice in a granary; they are always present, but in what number? Candida can be cultured in most people's blood, and it is so ubiquitous that it is usually ignored by microbiologists when they do come across it. The way to prove that a condition (or a cluster of conditions occurring together) is the result of Candida, is to treat it, and if the symptoms then disappear the proof is then irrefutable.

This is one of the very few instances where the treatment is in fact the main means of diagnosis. The initial suspicions that result in the treatment being applied, rely upon recognition of the sort of symptoms that might be implicated by the presence of Candida, as well as an awareness of those factors that influence Candida's development and behaviour. This knowledge, combined with a careful background history which looks at previous and current medical treatment and drug usage, as well as at diet and stress factors, will give clear indications as to the likelihood, or otherwise, of Candida being a possible culprit.

It is these areas that we are going to explore, in order to formulate a series of recommendations for the control of Candida, and for the prevention of its accompanying complications.

This exaggeration of a previously fairly harmless inter-action between ourselves and a yeast is one of the complications of civilization, and as such is rapidly becoming so widespread as to constitute an epidemic. The failure, thus far, by all but a handful of doctors to recognize the situation is tragic, for the degree of human suffering involved is enormous. Prevention is not difficult, and control, whilst a slow process, is not beyond the limits of any intelligent individual to institute.

The major credit for the unravelling of this mystery belongs to one man, who recognized that what he was seeing in his own patients had a worldwide import. He first set about diligently assembling his evidence, which he presented in a scientific journal (the *Journal of Ortho-molecular Psychiatry*). He then went back to his task of investigation. Over a period of years his results, in an enormous range of diseases, from acne to schizophrenia, and what appeared to be multiple sclerosis, were so impressive that in true fashion the world beat a path to his door. Dr C. Orion Truss, of Birmingham, Alabama, will be remembered for his work in this field by tens of thousands of grateful people. His masterly investigation and research, conducted in a normal medical practice, shows how important simple observation is in the quest for knowledge and the understanding of man's ills. Dr Truss has written his own history of this quest, and of the whole story of Candida, in his book, *The Missing Diagnosis*.

That book, and the excellent book on the same subject by another renowned American practitioner, Dr William Crook, entitled *The Yeast Connection*, both suggest for their attack on yeast, the use of an antifungal drug called nystatin. They also suggest other methods, including nutrition and desensitization. This book, however, will not attempt to echo the drug approach suggested by these two practitioners, but will present non-drug alter-natives to the use of nystatin. This is not to say that this drug should never be used – only that in most cases there are ways of restoring the competence of the body to fight the yeast itself. There are also naturally occurring nutrients which enhance the controlling of the wildly proliferating yeast. This is the only reason this book has needed to be written, for in every other way the two books mentioned above are excellent, and are valuable contributions to the literature of health.

Our task is now to look at the nature of the enemy, what makes it active, and what we must look for to recognize such activity. After that we will begin to learn how to deal with it.

2.

CANDIDA AND YOUR DEFENCE SYSTEM

The object of our interest is a member of the yeast family. Strictly speaking it is a member of a sub-group of that family of plants known as fungi (or moulds). Yeasts live practically everywhere on the planet. They can derive their nutrients from most organic sources. This means anything that is alive, or has been alive, can support yeasts. Rather than having roots like other plants, yeasts can derive their nutrients via the use of enzymes. Given the right conditions for growth and replication, yeast is capable of almost explosive growth, as anyone who has made bread will testify.

Roger Williams,[1] a world-renowned research scientist, states that if a single yeast cell is given a highly favourable environment, with a good assortment of nutrients, and the correct temperature, it can, within twenty-four hours, produce a colony of over a hundred yeast cells. At this rate of reproduction, Williams calculates, within one week, one cell could turn into a yeast colony weighing one billion tons. The fact that this has not happened, and that it is not likely to happen, is solely because the environment is seldom ideal for any creature on earth, least of all for yeast. It does, however, highlight a very pertinent point in our understanding of the Candida problem. Candida is a yeast which lives inside you and me, and, as far as is known, every other adult on earth, and most children as well. It seldom takes over our entire body, but when it does the consequences are horrific. It can only achieve such a state if the environment for it is excellent, and if the defence mechanisms that the body has with which to control its spread are weakened or absent.

As Williams points out, in nature, yeast cells are almost always hampered by imperfect or inadequate environmental conditions. Were it not so, they would have engulfed the earth long ago. Just the same fact controls the colonies of Candida (and other yeasts) that live in and on you.

Candida is usually a resident of your digestive system, largely in the intestines. It also tends to occupy sites in the vaginal regions and on the skin.

Research has shown that almost everyone has antibodies to Candida. This indicates that the individual's defence system has been challenged to respond to Candida's presence by producing antibodies. Truss states that by the age of six months, at the latest, Candida is living in or on at least 90 per cent of people, as evidenced by a positive skin test reaction when extracts of Candida are injected just under the skin.[2] This reaction shows that there has been a previous presence of the yeast to which the body has developed antibodies.

The fact that it is in all of us, and yet many people sail through life with no apparent ill effects, indicates that we have learned to cope with our passengers. Unlike certain other minute creatures that live in our digestive tract, and which serve a useful purpose, such as *lactobacillus acidophilus*, which helps with the breakdown of our foodstuff and helps in the synthesis of some of the B vitamins, there is no symbiotic relationship with Candida. There is no 'trade-off' whereby houseroom is given in exchange for some useful function. So Candida is a pure and simple parasite – a freeloading parasite. This is perhaps inevitable, in terms of the multitude of opportunistic microscopic creatures, of both the animal and vegetable kingdom. Most, if not all, plants and animals 'enjoy' similar relationships with bacteria and fungi. Some of these relationships are mutually beneficial and some are distinctly one-sided. So Candida, for all the musicality of its name, is an unwelcome boarder and a potential danger throughout life. Once we know just what sort of situations will remove our natural controls of it, and what will give it that extra ability to proliferate by virtue of an environment conducive to its growth, we will have the beginnings of a picture as to what needs to be done to contain it.

Part of this picture is indeed an understanding of the ways in which the body has learned to take care of the threat of parasites. It may be that we cannot actually stop it from taking up squatters' rights in our body, but we can certainly confine its activities to a small and relatively safe part of the premises.

We should try to understand some aspects of our body's amazing defensive capability. It has long been observed that people who survive certain infections seldom suffer from that same disease again. They develop antibodies to the infecting organism. Apart from conferring such specific resistance to various disease-causing microorganisms, the immune system plays a vital role in other biological reactions. We have, in essence, two systems, which together make up the immune system. One is based in the thymus gland (which lies just below your breast bone), which produces what are called T-cells. The other part of the immune system is made up of different types of white blood cells, called B-cells. These protect you from most bacterial invaders, and some viral infections. By producing molecules called antibodies, the B-cells neutralize many potential enemies. The two systems, together making up the surveillance and protection agency of the body, work in harmony, with, it is thought, the thymus taking the leading role.[3]

The white blood cells, which act as the soldiers in the front line of the battle, are manufactured mainly in the marrow of the long bones of the body. Some of these actually are turned into T-cells, by the influence of hormones from the thymus gland. Other white blood cells are turned into what are called lymphocytes. Anything that tries to get into the bloodstream, or the interior of the body, has to contend with the T- and B-cells, and their powerful ability to neutralize foreign substances or organisms. If a B-cell senses a foreign organism it produces antibodies that are specific against the invader. At the same time other B-cells are alerted to the alien presence, which causes them to manufacture antibodies to destroy the enemy.

It is believed that there are in excess of a million different kinds of antibodies in the bloodstream. As they are maufactured and deployed against the intruder, the lymphocytes go into action, with other white blood cells, to dispose of the debris and waste products of the battle between the intruder and the body. Thus a condition such as influenza is self-limiting, in that the fever and the symptoms of aching represent the intense body activity that is going on to deal with the invading virus, as well as the effects of the resulting degree of toxicity from the breakdown products of the battle.

When T-cells come across an invading organism, whether this be a virus or a fungus such as Candida (or even a mutant cancer cell), they produce what are called lymphokines which can kill micro-organisms (or cancer cells). One such lymphokine which has received much attention is interferon. Lymphokines can also call up assistance from a powerful ally in this battle called macrophage, which can eliminate micro-organisms and tumour cells by literally swallowing them whole. Sometimes the T-cells act as 'helper' cells to the B-cells in their production of antibodies to fight the invader, and they can also act as what are called 'suppressor' cells, to stop a defensive process from getting out of hand, when there may be a danger of B- or T-cells actually attacking friendly tissues in the body.

When for any one of a number of reasons (which we will consider in a later chapter) the immune system becomes weakened, we talk of the person being immuno-deficient, or of having a poor immune response. It is when these valiant soldiers, the T- and B-cells, and the macrophages and their various assistants are put into a weakened state, that silent squatters in our body can become free of the constraints that the defence system normally imposes, and spread to areas beyond their normal territory. At that point a vast array of problems and symptoms can arise.

This system of defence, with its checks and balances, may become disrupted to such an extent that the condition now known simply by its initials, AIDS, may occur. The initials stand for Acquired Immuno-Deficiency Syndrome, and in this condition it is the T-cells (from the thymus gland) that function inadequately. In fact the ratio between the helper and suppressor cells alters so that there is an excess of suppressor cells, in contrast with the opposite situation in normal health. One research effort in the AIDS battle involves the use of thymosin, a hormone produced by the thymus. It is obviously desirable to enhance the function of the thymus gland so that it can produce adequate, active T-cells and the desired amount of hormone. Among the nutrient factors which we can use to this end are vitamin C and the amino acid arginine. The amounts used in treating conditions, such as AIDS, where the immune system is severely disrupted are very large indeed (upwards of 20g of vitamin C daily, and 3-5g of arginine).

When the immune system is in a weakened state, not only do infections become more frequent but severe consequences arise, such as greater likelihood of cancer developing, because of the reduced surveillance by the B- and T-cells. In such a condition of inadequate protection it is no wonder that the ever-present opportunistic yeast may slip through the defence barrier and advance to areas previously closed to it. This is a simplistic picture of what happens, but it contains the essential facts. It is known that before it becomes invasive, the yeast (Candida) alters to a different form, known as its mycelial fungal form, in which it has characteristics which make it more dangerous, such as a root structure enabling it to penetrate through the mucosal barriers, with a variety of harmful consequences (see Chapter 4).

Recent research by Dr Truss[35] indicates that many of the toxic effects noted with Candida activity result from its ability to manufacture, under appropriate conditions, the substance acetaldehyde. He points out that this well-known toxin could produce both the clinical and the laboratory characteristics of Candida infection. He has analysed the amino acid profiles of the affected individuals in order to arrive at this finding and maintains that this theory appeals because it defines the symptoms of chronic yeast infection in terms of a toxin which common strains of Candida can be shown to produce in laboratory conditions. This provides the chemical link between normal yeast fermentation and the metabolic abnormalities found in susceptible patients. He stresses that no conclusive proof yet exists that Candida can ferment sugar into acetaldehyde in the body, but that this is highly probable, based on the evidence thus far.

There is also evidence from a variety of sources[36, 37, 38] that there is a degree of immune system depression which results from mercury toxicity reaching the body via amalgam fillings in the teeth. A number of researchers have shown there are several ways in which this highly toxic metal is able to penetrate into the body, and that this has a specific harmful effect on the immune system. There is evidence that this can be linked with the spread of Candida activity. A number of dentists are now helping affected individuals by removing mercury amalgams and replacing them with either a composite or gold filling. It should be stressed that research into the relationship between mercury, derived from amalgam fillings, and health problems in general and Candida involvement in particular, is as yet incomplete. That there is a link seems probable, however, and it is worth considering alternative choices for the filling of teeth, other than amalgams which contain mercury. The replacement of existing fillings may be required in cases where a link can be demonstrated between the health status and measurable mercury toxicity resulting from amalgams. The use of amino acid compounds, such as Glutathione, and of vitamin C, can help to ease mercury deposits from the body. Tests can be done to measure the sensitivity of the body to mercury, and also to measure the levels of mercury in the mouth (escaping as a gas), as well as the electrical activity in the teeth, set up by the combinations of metals in the mouth. These methods, as well as measuring mercury levels via hair analysis, can all indicate just how active this problem is in any particular individual.

Our ultimate attempt to neutralize and control the spread and effects of Candida (for we can seldom get rid of it completely) depends upon the use of whatever safe methods we have at our disposal, to deprive it of its ideal nutrients, whilst at the same time building up, and enhancing, the embarrassed and depleted immune system. This can then get on with the job of keeping Candida in check. It is this double thrust of activity which we must undertake if we are to do more than temporarily suppress Candida. The use of an antifungal drug will, it is true, in time destroy a great deal of Candida's potency and reduce its resultant symptoms. However, this will stop happening the moment the drug is stopped. The answer to controlling Candida in the long term lies in a two-pronged attack which deprives the yeast of its optimum nutrient environment, as well as the reinstitution of normal controls, via the immune system and healthy intestinal flora. As we will see, there are other methods which, it is thought, can help by altering the ability of the yeast to multiply, and we will consider these natural, safe alternatives to the use of drugs later.

It must, however, be stated that there are conditions in which the use of antifungal drugs are to be advocated, especially if the condition is such as to indicate that the process of recovery is going to be a very long one. In the main, however, once we can learn to recognize those symptoms that indicate Candida getting out of hand, the natural, non-drug methods that I am suggesting will work, and work well. Nystatin is the main such antifungal drug now in use. Whilst effective against certain Candida strains, others are resistant to it. Not being a broad spectrum antifungal agent it allows proliferation of other fungi, such as trichophyton, when Candida is attacked.[39] An alternative exists in caprylic acid, an extract of coconuts (see page 77).

We will now go on to consider just what can happen to weaken your wonderful defence mechanism, the immune system, as well as additional ways in which Candida is sometimes allowed to go on the rampage, and so begin to infest other areas of your body.

3.

HOW CANDIDA GETS OUT OF HAND

There are a number of predisposing factors which will allow Candida to get wildly out of control. To a greater or lesser extent these same factors may be involved in the more subtle spread of Candida which represents what happens in the majority of people affected by the sort of symptoms outlined in Chapter 1. There is a degree of overlap of course, for seldom will only one factor be involved. Among the main ones are:

1. An underlying inherited or acquired deficiency of the immune system.
2. The aftermath of steroids (hormones) in food or as medication.
3. The aftermath of antibiotics in food or as medication.
4. Diabetes.

As we shall see, these factors are also vitally interconnected with the diet of the individual, which 'feeds' the yeast. We will look at each of these and see how they transform Candida from its relatively docile state into that of a predator. First let us consider ways in which the immune system can be weakened.

Immune System Deficiency

As we have seen in the previous chapter, part of the response of the body to an intruder such as Candida is the production of antibodies to meet the particular antigen (a substance which stimulates a response on the part of the immune system) that is present in the foreign substance or organism. Candida has many antigens, and the efficiency with which the defensive operation is carried out, against any particular one of these antigens, can to some extent be inborn (i.e. genetic). There is a great variation in the degree of response in any one person to the different antigens. This can lead to a situation in which the immune system, unable to adequately counteract and expel the Candida invasion, tolerates it in increasing amounts.

It has been demonstrated by research that we are all biochemically individual. [4, 5] This means that there are wide variations in the particular requirements for any of the over forty nutrients that we require for survival and health. Many of these individual needs are determined before birth, and this has led to the genetotrophic theory of disease causation. This, put simply, says that because a person has individual inborn requirements, which may vary greatly from a mythical 'average' or 'normal' amount, there is a good chance of one or other of these needs not being met by the normal dietary intake. This leads at best to a lowered degree of function, and at worst to a deficiency disease.

To a large extent this individual inborn (genetic) factor also applies to our ability to handle one or other of the pathogens, or micro-organisms, capable of infecting us. This is the case in our ability to handle Candida efficiently. It seems that since infestation by this yeast is almost universal, we are incapable of totally controlling its presence in our bodies. Some people will be more able than others to keep it under control, and limit its spread. Thus some people will, without the involvement of such factors as antibiotics and steroid drugs (see below), become 'tolerant' of a degree of spread of the yeast.

The commonest areas for this spread to occur are in the mouth, the throat and in the vaginal areas. If this initially produces a degree of reaction and activity on behalf of the immune system, then we would see manifestations of the condition called thrush. This would flare up periodically when, perhaps, there were factors which lowered the general vitality. Eventually, in many cases, the condition might no longer evoke an acute flare-up, but would remain in a semi-permanent, chronic state. This happens when the body becomes 'tolerant' of the yeast's 'foothold', and is no longer able to mount attacks on it. This is an indication of impaired or deficient immune function. Among the many aspects of our environment which can influence this are stress factors, nutritional inadequacy and pollution, as well as the use of specific drugs which weaken the immune system further.

We are all nowadays familiar with the concept of tissue and organ transplantation. This involves the use of powerful drugs which are designed to prevent the body of the recipient from rejecting the new foreign tissue or organ. These are called immuno-suppressive drugs, simply because it is their prime task to stop the natural defences from working adequately – in other words, to suppress the immune system. The risk of infection and of other diseases resulting from this is all too familiar to patients who have gone through such treatment. Drugs such as steroids (hormones) have this effect, and these are employed in a variety of conditions ranging from rheumatic disorders to asthma and hormonal imbalances. The most widespread use of steroids, however, is not in the treatment of disease but in the contraceptive pill. One of the most devastating effects of the long-term use of this type of medication is on the immune system in general, and on the ability of Candida to proliferate wildly, in particular.

The contraceptive pill is dealt with more fully below.

There are now known to be a variety of nutrient substances which are absolutely vital for the adequate functioning of the immune system.[6, 7] These include a number of vitamin and mineral substances which have antioxidant properties. This means that they are able to slow down, or stop, a process in which substances known as 'free radicals' can cause tissue damage. The major free-radical scavengers are vitamin C, vitamin E (acting in conjunction with a substance called selenium) as well as certain amino acids (parts of the protein chain) such as methionine, cysteine and glutathione (which is itself a combination of three amino acids – cysteine, glutamic acid and glycine). Vitamin B6 (pyridoxine), zinc, manganese and other important nutrients have been shown to be involved in compromising the immune system when deficient.[8]

It should be realized that apart from the nutrients mentioned in this section, it is possible for any of the forty-plus nutrients vital to life to be required in extra-ordinary amounts by a particular person to meet idiosyncratic inborn needs. These needs may also vary markedly under different conditions (infection, stress, pregnancy, etc.) in the same person, and so any vitamin, mineral or other nutrient, is capable of upsetting the chain of complex biochemical interactions which allow the immune function to operate efficiently. The ones cited above just happen to have a more dramatic impact than some of the others. Assessment of personal needs is a task requiring patience. Some personal detective work can be useful, and books such as *Your Personal Health Programme* by Jeffrey Bland (Thorsons) and *Your Personal Vitamin Profile* by Michael Colgan (Blond & Briggs) enable this to be successfully achieved by using questionnaires aimed at providing specific indications as to nutrient requirements.

Stress, which involves repeated, or constant, states of

anxiety, and all that this entails in terms of depletion of
vital nutrient reserves, as well as imbalances of internal
secretions and functions, is a major cause of immune
incompetence. One of the ways in which this can be most
dramatically demonstrated is that during periods of stress
people become far more prone to infection. This indicates
the lowered efficiency of their immune system, as well as
the increased usage by the body of vital nutrients such as
zinc and vitamin C at such times.

The interaction between anxiety/stress conditions and
nutritional incompetence leads to the immune system
being deprived of the ability to operate efficiently. If at
the same time there is increased demand on the effective
functioning of the immune system, to meet environmental
or nutritional toxicity (pollution of air, cigarette smoke,
alcohol, caffeine-rich drinks such as coffee, chocolate and
tea) then a complex picture emerges in which excessive
demands, inadequate nutrition (with associated deficiencies)
and perhaps drug usage, such as the contraceptive pill, all
interact to deplete the immune function. Let us examine
the manner in which drugs in common use can further
complicate the situation.

Antibiotics, 'the Pill' and Steroids

It is clear from many years of research that the use of
antibiotics removes from the scene biological controls
over the yeast that lives in us. As has been mentioned, one
of the major sites for this to take place is the long, dark,
warm and moist (ideal environment for yeast) digestive
tract, which it should be noted is also inhabited by
upwards of 5lb of other micro-organisms, most of which
are friendly and helpful to the body. One such friend is
Lactobacillus acidophilus, which by its presence helps to
keep a check on the spread of yeast. When antibiotics are
used to destroy pathogenic (harmful) micro-organisms
which might be harming the body (as in treating an

infection), the friendly bacteria in the bowel are also destroyed, or severely damaged. When this occurs, the yeast, which is totally unaffected by the antibiotic (being a yeast and not a bacteria), will find room for expansion. This becomes even more likely as the resistance of the immune system will at that time be compromised. In a variety of ways the same thing happens with the use of steroid drugs, such as cortisone (even cortisone ointments, so commonly prescribed for skin problems cause a yeast increase, by being absorbed into the system). All steroids, including those used in the contraceptive pill, will have a depressing effect on the immune system.

It is worth noting at this point that there is another, almost totally ignored source of antibiotics and hormonal residues, to which all but the vegetarian sector of the population are exposed. This is of course commercially reared meat and poultry (with the exception of lamb). Antibiotics and hormones are fed to animals in order to speed their growth as well as to control the heightened susceptibility to disease that their unnatural existence generates.

Anyone who has been regularly eating beef, pork, veal and chicken (and many people eat one or more of these daily) will have absorbed prodigious amounts of antibiotic and hormone residues (unless the source of the meat was from a farm which did not employ the addition of such drugs).

Low-level intake of these substances over many years may have a devastating effect on the ability to control Candida, as would the regular employment of these drugs in the form of medications. This area is yet to be adequately researched, but it does provide one more argument in favour of adopting a vegetarian diet.

It has also been noted that, because of the hormonal changes that take place during pregnancy, a degree of control over Candida is lost. Yeast therefore finds this a good time to expand its activities.

Imagine then, if you will, a young lady who has grown up in this era characterized by common usage of these drugs. She has had antibiotics prescribed to her over the years for minor problems such as tonsillitis and ear infection. She may have then developed cystitis from time to time, and also have had a broad-spectrum antibiotic for this.Her skin may have had a good deal of acne, and again this would commonly have been attacked with antibiotics. Should she have had cause, she may have had steroids for asthma or some other condition. Going on 'the Pill', and subsequently coming off it and becoming pregnant, would also have enhanced the chances of yeast spreading, and causing problems (the acne and cystitis are frequent examples of Candida activity). Thus the child in her womb would be exposed to a variety of antigens (up to 790) from the Candida activity in her body, all the while inheriting the possibility of a weak immune response (not all children inherit a weak response), and so the pattern will be set to repeat itself. We have still left out of this picture all the other variables, such as nutritional imbalances, which are common in modern society: pollution; excessive use of sugar-rich foods (which yeast loves), and stress factors in general. The picture emerges of a person who is doing just about all that is possible to bring about the ideal conditions for yeast to thrive in. And the result, in terms of the general population, of this typical scenario? An explosion of Candida-caused problems, over the past thirty years or so, which is now reaching epidemic proportions.

We will discuss later a very important aspect of Candida's spread, which is the diet of the individual, not in the sense of helping to create a situation in which the immune system is less efficient, but as adding actual supporting nutrients to Candida. The two main areas in which this occurs are the use of sugar-rich foods, which all yeasts love, as well as foods that are themselves associated with yeasts or fungi. In the meantime it should be evident that many aspects of life in civilized society are working towards the disadvantage or our defensive ability, and to the advantage of prospective enemies, such as Candida.

Dr Truss, who has done so much to research and publicize the Candida problem, is scathing in his attack on the use of certain drugs which have compounded the problem. Antibiotics are often used inadvisedly, in cases in which they have no role to play at all. Incorrectly diagnosed viral and fungal conditions may be uselessly treated by antibiotics, for example. This actually increases the likelihood of the condition worsening. The treatment of acne with tetracycline is another major cause of Candida spreading, and Truss insists that there is no way anyone suffering from Candida problems can control their condition if they continue with tetracycline. In many cases acne is actually the direct result of Candida infection, and will worsen rather than improve on such treatment.

In the use of the contraceptive hormone, too, Truss sees great harm. Fully 35 per cent of women using the Pill have, associated with it, acute vaginal candidiasis. There are undoubtedly many others who have less pronounced changes in this regard, as their immune competence is gradually compromised by the hormonal onslaught. As Truss points out, 'Chronic yeast vaginitis tends to be at its worst when progesterone levels are high, as in pregnancy, and the luteal phase of the menstrual cycle. Therefore the progesterone component of contraceptive hormones may well be responsible for their effect.' It is clear that the association between Candida vaginitis and emotional problems such as irritability and depression frequently appears soon after the first use of the contraceptive pill. It is worth reflecting on the fact that the degree of biological individuality which we display in our individual reactions to any harmful factor such as Candida must play a large part in deciding just who will, and who will not, succumb to a spread of Candida. Since 35 per cent of women do not control the vaginal Candida when on the Pill, we must assume that the other 65 per cent do. This highlights the fact that for many people there is an inborn genetic weakness in their ability to meet such a challenge. For some this will have been acquired via the very factors we have been discussing in this chapter – antibiotics, immune system weakened by stress, nutritional factors, etc. We shall see that the approach to controlling Candida must include methods that deal both with the building up of the immune system, as well as reducing as many factors as possible which help to sustain the yeast in its advance. Among the most important of these is the eliminating of the use (unless absolutely vital) of antibiotics, hormone preparations and contraceptive pills, as well as the making of alterations in the diet to avoid actually feeding the yeast.

Since yeast loves sugar, it is clear that if a person has additional levels of sugar in the bloodstream, as in a diabetic condition, this will fuel the spread of Candida. For this reason diabetic individuals are more prone than average to Candida problems, and they must be even more rigorous in their efforts to control it.

The possible involvement of mercury toxicity in harming immune system control of Candida has been mentioned (see page 21) and deserves re-emphasis.

Foods that Help to Spread Candida

Yeast loves carbohydrate-rich foods. This in effect means that we must attempt to deprive it of its sustenance by limiting, or cutting out all together, all sugar-rich foods and refined carbohydrates. Details of this will be outlined in the nutritional programme (Chapter 5). It is also considered to be important that the intake of any foods that contain fermented products, moulds or fungi be limited.[2, 9] This means things such as vinegar, alcoholic beverages, yeast extracts and spreads, mushrooms, blue cheeses. This aspect of the programme to control Candida should be carefully observed at the outset. Once the yeast is controlled, there is no reason to keep to a strict prohibition, but the return of classic symptoms of Candida activity, such as abdominal bloating after eating one of the offending foods, will tell you if it is time to return for a period to the avoidance strategy. Just as foods which contain moulds or fungi are considered undesirable, so will it be found that symptoms will always be worse in humid, damp environments, which are conducive to mould and fungus spores being present in the atmosphere. Thus, it is important to eliminate from the home any areas of damp on walls, etc., as many moulds can reinforce the effects of Candida by their presence. For this reason, inhaled spores of any mould or fungus should be avoided during the active phase of Candida infection.

Candida gets out of hand because we allow it to. We may well do so in ignorance, but it is folly to blame the yeast when we have the power to control it, as millions of people have done before. Once you begin to suspect that your many and varied symptoms (see next chapter) may be the result of Candida activity, it is time to grasp the problem firmly and take responsibility for the situation. Candida will not go away. Its current spree may be the result of any combination of factors which have released it from our normal efficient control. To get it back where it belongs (or at least to where it can do least harm) we must restore our defence capacity to its optimum, and we must stop doing those things that are helping the yeast to thrive. It's as simple as that. You can do this by your own efforts, by the reform of your dietary pattern, by the use of particular nutrient substances, and by overall stress and pollution reduction. Once you have put Candida in its place, you can relax your vigilance to a great extent, in the sense of allowing your diet to contain certain of the 'undesirable' substances from time to time, but you should be aware of the factors which allow Candida to advance in the first place, and avoid these as stringently as possible.

We will now look at the sort of problems that Candida can cause when it gets out of control. Be prepared for some surprises.

4.

CANDIDA AND ITS CONSEQUENCES TO YOUR HEALTH

The actual list of conditions in which Candida has been implicated as a major causative factor is very long indeed.

As has been mentioned, it is necessary to deduce the involvement of Candida from the history of the patient. (Were antibiotics used? Is, or was, the contraceptive pill in use? Have cortisones or other steroids, e.g. prednisone, been employed? etc.) The range and type of symptoms also give indications of its involvement. This is because it is useless asking a microbiology lab to look for Candida's presence, since we already know it to be present in practically all adults. So what would an analysis prove? We must deduce from the history and the symptoms that Candida seems to be involved. The proof of its involvement is obtained by carrying out an anti-Candida programme and finding out whether or not this gets rid of most of the list of symptoms usually present.

Before considering them all (or at least the major ones) one by one, let us look at a list of the sort of conditions that are now known to be the possible result of Candida's activity.

Vaginitis; thrush (oral or vaginal); endometriosis; athlete's foot; headaches (migraine type); fatigue; constipation;

bloating; allergy; sensitivity to perfumes, fumes, chemical odours and tobacco smoke; poor memory, feelings of unreality, irritability, inability to concentrate; depression; numbness, tingling and weak muscles; heart-burn; abdominal pain; diarrhoea; recurrent sore throats and nasal congestion; swelling and discomfort in joints; blurred vision, and so on – and on. The diagnosis becomes more clear if symptoms are aggravated during damp weather (or places) or when in an environment with a lot of mould or fungus. Also, if the symptoms are worse after eating sugar-rich or fungus-containing foods, the evidence for Candida's involvement becomes stronger.

After we have looked at these conditions more closely, we will try to put all this together in the form of a questionnaire, which should enable you to assess the chances of Candida being involved in your health make-up. Truss draws a picture of a typical case of chronic Candida infection in his article 'Restoration of Immuno-logical Competence to Candida Albicans'.[10] He states, after pointing to the influence of multiple pregnancies, birth control pills, antibiotics and cortisone, as well as other factors that depress the immune system:

The onset of local symptoms of yeast infection, in relation to the use of these drugs, is especially significant and usually precedes the systemic response. Repeated courses of antibiotics and birth-control pills, often punctuated with multiple pregnancies, lead to ever increasing symptoms of mucosal infections in the vagina and gastro-intestinal tract. Accompanying these are manifestations of tissue injury, based on immuno-logical and possibly toxic responses to yeast products released into the systemic circulation. Many infections are secondary to allergic responses of the mucous membranes of the respiratory tract, urethra and bladder, necessitating increasingly frequent antibiotic therapy that simultaneously aggravates, and perpetuates, the underlying cause of the allergic membrane, that allowed the infection. Depression is common, often associated with difficulty in memory, reasoning and concentration. These symptoms are especially severe in women, who in addition have great difficulty with the explosive irritability, crying and loss of self-confidence that are so characteristic of abnormal function of the ovarian hormones.

Truss then points out that accompanying this sad catalogue are what he calls 'poor end-organ response' resulting in acne; loss of libido (disinterest in sex); menstrual bleeding and cramps; intolerance to foods and chemicals, etc. The commonest (but by no means only) type of individual suffering from Candida infection, is seen to be a woman somewhere between puberty and the menopause, who has undergone some, or all, of the predisposing factors described previously, and who has some, or all, of the symptoms outlined in Truss's picture above. A mixture of unaccountable vaginal and bowel symptoms, ranging from discharge and itching, to bloating, discomfort, diarrhoea and/or constipation; as well as an array of mental-emotional symptoms are typical. Classically such women are labelled as neurotic, and this must be the crowning insult to an individual who has literally begun to feel her body and mind giving way in all directions.

The vaginal and intestinal tracts are the most usual areas for Candida to inhabit, since they provide the damp atmosphere, and the nutrients it thrives on. If circumstances allow, Candida has been known to spread along the entire length of the digestive tract, from the anus to the mouth. The tongue may be coated, and there may be yeast deposits on the insides of the cheeks, the corners of the mouth and gums. White spots and a coating on the tongue are the obvious signs, accompanied by a soreness and tingling of the gums. When the oesophagus is affected it can result in symptoms commonly assigned to 'heartburn'; indigestion and acid stomach are symptoms which can be the result of Candida activity in the stomach region. If the infestation is prolific in the small or large intestine, then diarrhoea may be the result. This may be chronic, and may be accompanied by mucus and/or blood. There may be cramp-like pains ('spastic colon') and colicky pains, often associated with difficulty in passing normal bowel motions. Bloating and distension of the abdomen is a frequent occurrence with Candida, and there may be a variety of abdominal noises as a result. If constipation is indeed a factor, then haemorrhoids are a likely consequence, as is the possibility of rectal discomfort and itching.

The very nature of Candida changes under certain conditions. It can turn into what is called its 'mycelial fungal' form, from its simple yeast form. Candida is what is known as a dimorphic organism. This means that it has two quite separate identities. In the yeast form it has no root, but in its fungal form it produces what are called rhizoids. These are long structures, similar to roots. The complication that this presents is that these 'roots' can actually penetrate through the mucosa of the tissue in which they are growing. Thus the boundary between the body proper, and the self-contained world of the digestive tract, can be breached. This allows substances to enter the bloodstream of the individual which would otherwise have been kept out by this boundary. The fungal form of the Candida organism is invasive, and it can use this avenue to enter the body proper. The main result of the breaking of the intestinal barrier is that undigested proteins from the food eaten, as well as toxic wastes from the Candida infestation, may begin to circulate in the bloodstream. These are frequently the cause of a wide variety of disseminated symptoms, often of an allergic type. If these substances reach the brain, there is a chance for the production of what have been termed 'brain allergies'.[11] These can result in a wide variety of mood and personality problems, ranging from depression, irritability and mood swings, to conditions which look for all the world like the symptoms of schizophrenia.

These substances, which enter the brain and act upon the receptors there, to produce these mental and personality symptoms, have been given the label *exorphins*.[12] This differentiates them from *endorphins*, which are substances produced in the body which have roles to play in the control of many aspects of the biochemistry of life, including pain control. The externally originating substances (proteins from incompletely digested food) which slip into the bloodstream through the gates opened by fungal 'roots' of Candida are able to cause havoc in whatever tissues they come into contact with. They will be seen as 'foreign' by the immune system, which will attempt to neutralize them. If such a process is long continued, and this sort of thing can run on for many years, then this in itself is a factor contributing to the ultimate depletion of the immune function of the body. It simply becomes overwhelmed by the constant onslaught. The defensive reaction by the immune system to such substances may result in a wide range of what are seen as allergic symptoms, including asthmatic attacks, nasal and respiratory conditions, skin reactions, palpitations, aches and swellings, etc.

The female reproductive organs are a major site for Candida activity. If it irritates the urethra it can be a common cause of cystitis. If, for any of a number of reasons, the acidity of the region alters, then the relatively benign yeast form can alter into the fungal form, and become actively invasive and spread to other regions, accessible from the vagina. This can lead to inflammatory conditions in the womb, fallopian tubes and ovaries themselves (see Chapter 7, 'Case Histories'). A wide variety of consequences can be envisaged, including the tragic possibility of infertility or sterility. The symptoms related to Candida involvement in this region can range from frequency of urination, coupled with a burning sensation, to chronic discharge, as well as pre-menstrual and menstrual problems, and the whole gamut of inflammatory and infectious involvements of the reproductive system.

The concurrence of mild, or major, emotional and mental symptoms with any such pattern of ill health should alert you to the strong possibility of Candida activity. Often mental symptoms are no more than a general feeling of inability to concentrate, accompanied by memory lapses, and feelings of lethargy and exhaustion. They may, however, be far more dramatic, as Truss and others have proved. The first articles on the subject, by Truss, discussed the fact that many conditions are given names or 'labels' simply because they fit into a pattern which is more or less recognizable as being similar to a particular known illness. That is to say, a combination of symptoms which may have no obvious cause, is somehow more 'manageable' medically if it is labelled.

Truss initially reported on six cases. Two of these women had been repeatedly diagnosed as 'schizophrenic'. Another woman in this original report was diagnosed previously as having 'multiple sclerosis'. Pointing out that they all recovered on anti-yeast treatment, and that they were all in good health up to seventeen years after recovery, he asks the pertinent question, 'Were two of these women really schizophrenic, or was it just that *Candida albicans* was responsible for brain function so abnormal that highly competent specialists never doubted the diagnosis of schizophrenia?'. He further asks, 'In the third woman, did *Candida albicans* induce neurological abnormalities sufficiently typical of multiple sclerosis that a competent neurologist would mistakedly diagnose the disease?' He answers by saying that either the treatment dealt with a yeast infection, which can produce symptoms which mimic these diseases (and many others) or that yeast can actually cause the diseases which are labelled with these names. The indication, after many years of work by Truss and others, is that this is not just a case of remission (which is not uncommon in either schizophrenia or multiple sclerosis) but that Candida induces symptoms *similar* to those of other illnesses, which may then be wrongly diagnosed and labelled.

It is clear that the ramifications of Candida infection are not yet fully understood, and that much clarification and research remains to be done. In the meantime, since it is not difficult to identify reasons to suspect its possible involvement, it seems reasonable that a Candida-control approach should be adopted in cases where the history and symptoms approximate any of the patterns touched on above, whatever previous diagnosis has been made. The treatment is, after all, harmless and indeed health-promoting. Other conditions which are sometimes confused with Candida involvement are frequently labelled as psychosomatic. This can be a way for the doctor to avoid having to say that he cannot find the cause. Calling conditions such as this 'functional' or 'psychosomatic' may, if repeated, result in patients beginning to believe the they really *are* not quite balanced. The terms 'neurotic' and 'nervous' are often ascribed to such individuals, with devastating effects on morale and self-esteem. The yeast or fungal cause may remain unsuspected or, if noted as part of the problem (if thrush is a part of the 'psychosomatic' symptom picture for example), be simply ignored as a minor piece of the puzzle, unworthy of therapeutic effort.

There is reason to believe that Candida infection is a rampant problem in modern society. It has been let loose by the use of drugs, used in good faith to help in other directions, as well as by a dietary pattern which is ideal for the sustenance of the yeast, rather than the host. The number and variety of possible consequences is mind-boggling and deserves the attention of every individual involved in the healing professions.

The alertness of one man has brought about the current increase in awareness of the significance of Candida. He may not be totally right in his concept, but the results he has so far obtained in thousands of cases bearing a range of symptoms such as those already discussed – simply by paying attention to the yeast component of the problem – are proof of the validity of this method of treatment.

There is no area of health more amenable to self-assessment and self-help, and the information which will be provided in subsequent chapters should enable improvement in most cases in which Candida is the culprit.

The questionnaires on the following pages will give you the chance to assess the possibility of Candida being a major part of your current health picture. It is possible for most of the symptoms described to be the result of causes other than Candida. If, however, you have more than one of the indications on List 2, as well as some of the lesser symptoms listed at the end of the questionnaire, then the possibility increases to a probability, especially if you can identify a possible causative link with at least one of the factors in List 1.

Candida Albicans Checklist
The completion of this questionnaire will give clues as to whether Candida is an active agent in your current health spectrum. It is not possible to make a diagnosis by these means alone, but a strong indication, as evidenced by positive answers in all sections of the questionnaire, is

possible and can be used to assist in deciding upon the undertaking of the Candida control programme.

List 1 – History of Drug Usage, etc
1. Have you ever taken a course of antibiotics for an infectious condition which lasted for either eight weeks or longer, or for short periods four or more times in one year?

2. Have you ever taken a course of antibiotics for the treatment of acne for a month or more continuously?

3. Have you ever had a course of steroid treatment such as predisone, cortisone or ACTH?

4. Have you ever taken contraceptive medication for a year or more?

5. Have you ever been treated with immuno-suppressant drugs?

6. Have you been pregnant more than once?

List 2 – Major Symptom History (Candida Implicated)
1. Have you in the past had recurrent or persistent cystitis, vaginitis or prostatis?

2. Have you a history of endometriosis?

3. Have you had thrush (oral or vaginal) more than once?

4. Have you ever had athlete's foot or a fungal infection of the nails or skin?

5. Are you severely affected by exposure to chemical fumes, perfumes, tobacco smoke, etc.? Or are your symptoms worse after taking yeasty or sugary foods or drinks?

6. Do you suffer from a variety of allergies?

7. Do you commonly suffer from abdominal distension, 'bloating', diarrhoea or constipation?

8. Do you suffer from pre-menstrual syndrome (fluid retention, irritability, etc)?

9. Do you suffer from depression, fatigue, lethargy, poor memory, feelings of 'unreality'?

10. Do you crave for sweet foods, bread or alcohol?

11. Do you suffer from unaccountable muscle aches, tingling, numbness or burning?

12. Do you suffer from unaccountable aches and swelling in joints?

13. Do you have vaginal discharge or irritation, or menstrual cramp or pain?

14. Do you have erratic vision or spots before the eyes?

15. Do you suffer from impotence or lack of sexual desire?

If there are one or more positive answers to the first section, and two or more in the second section, as well as some of the following being present, then Candida is probably involved in your symptoms causation. Symptoms usually worse on damp days; persistent drowsiness; lack of co-ordination; headaches; mood swings; loss of balance; rashes; mucus in stools; belching and 'wind'; bad breath; dry mouth; post-nasal drip; nasal itch and/or congestion; nervous irritability; tightness in chest; dry mouth or throat; ear sensitivity or fluid in ears; heartburn and indigestion.

5.

CONTROLLING CANDIDA NATURALLY (INCLUDING SUPPLEMENT PROGRAMME AND DIET)

If it has been possible to come to a position where it looks as though Candida is a likely suspect in your condition, then it is necessary to prove this by means of adopting an anti-Candida programme. If this succeeds in making a major impact upon your condition, by virtue of its controlling Candida and improving your symptom picture, then you will have proved the assumption to be correct. Dr W. M. Crook calls this a 'therapeutic trial'.[9] It is really the only way of being sure, since there is as yet no way of discovering whether Candida is involved by any laboratory tests.

This is a stumbling block for many people. They want cast-iron 'proof' that Candida is the culprit. Nonetheless all we can do is look at the picture that is currently present in your particular condition and add to this a review of your past history. If that looks like a 'Candida picture', then there really is no other choice but to introduce anti-Candida measures, apart from going on as you are. If a culture were made of your fluid discharges, tissues or excreta, it would inevitably display Candida's presence, somewhere in your body. This would not prove or disprove anything, as far as your symptoms are concerned, since a positive test result could also be obtained from almost every adult in the land. Only by looking at the known and suspected pattern of symptom production that has been built up around Candida's activity can we guess its active presence (as opposed to its benign presence if your immune system and intestinal flora are keeping it under control). The only real proof is in the treatment results. If you are better after controlling Candida, then you will know that what you assumed was accurate, and that your programme was the correct one. The very least that you will achieve is that you will have reformed your dietary pattern, and will have swallowed some harmless vitamins and other supplements, as well as building up your immune system's ability to combat its adversaries.

The controlling of Candida falls into three different segments. First there are a number of nutrient supplements which, for several reasons, can help to control Candida. Secondly there is a pattern of eating which reduces the intake of yeast-conducive foods and so deprives it of its growth potential. Finally there are specialized methods and substances, including antifungal drugs, which can be employed only by a health professional. These will be described to complete the picture of anti-Candida methods, although, as has been stressed, it is in the self-help field that the greatest long-term results will be found, and the first two segments of the programme, special supplements and diet, will prove to be worthy of adoption by anyone suspicious of Candida's role in their current health picture.

There are also a number of general tips which can be useful in coming to terms with the condition, and these will be found at the end of this chapter.

Specialized Supplemental Anti-Candida Methods
When antibiotics are used they destroy a number of

'friendly' bacteria which inhabit the digestive tract, and which, as well as providing other valuable symbiotic (mutually beneficial) contributions to the body's economy, also act as a controlling element, in stopping Candida from spreading. One of the major bacterial 'friends' which we have is *Lactobacillus acidophilus*. If sufficient of this bacteria can be encouraged to re-establish residence in the bowel, it will push back the yeast, which may have crowded into the vacant space left when antibiotics destroyed acidophilus colonies. *Lactobacillus acidophilus* is obtainable in a number of forms. It comes in capsules, and also in its active state in some yogurt cultures. Cultured milk products containing acidophilus should therefore play a part in the anti-Candida programme. The taking of acidophilus is also an important element in this programme.

There are variations on the source and type of acidophilus which are worth mentioning. A recent development in the USA is the introduction of 'Megadophilus' (marketed in the UK as 'Superdophilus'). There are over 200 strains of *Lactobacillus acidophilus* and one in particular has been identified by a research authority in the field of cultured dairy produce, Natasha Trenev, as being infinitely more potent in its ability to destroy other bacteria, than others. This has been incorporated into 'Megadophilus', which contains at least one billion active organisms, per gram. This is over a hundred times more potent than comparable commercial acidophilus preparations, and, in some cases, many thousands of times more potent. This and another similar product, 'Vital Dophilus', should be the first choices in acidophilus supplementation. (See 'Further Information' for suppliers.) Dosage of Superdophilus or Vital Dophilus, if as dry powder or as a capsule, is 2g (or 1 teaspoonful) three times daily between meals. If available as a powder the acidophilus should be kept refrigerated, and never exposed to temperatures above 80°F/27°C.

Dosages of up to 10g daily are in order (5 teaspoonsful of powder) with no toxic level known. When consumed as a powder, it should be stirred into non-chilled water, and drunk. This is best done well away from mealtimes. The acidophilus culture will become active in the small intestine, where it produces a number of nutritional compounds, including lactic acid, B-vitamins and enzymes, as well as natural antibiotic compounds.[13, 14, 15]

It may not be realized, but in the average bowel there exist colonies of micro-organisms which in total weight come to between 3 and 5 lb. These are not all helpful or friendly, and in order to repopulate the bowel with such helpful residents as acidophilus, large amounts are required. In re-establishing their territorial claim, the intruders such as Candida will be pushed back and often eliminated from the area.

Some researchers have found that acidophilus cultured on human milk is more effective than that which uses animal milk, and this technique is believed to be that used in the manufacture of Megadophilus. (See 'Further Information' for supplier.)[16]

This then is the first of the anti-Candida supplements you should introduce, together with acidophilus-cultured yogurt and/or sour milk with meals. The next major nutrient employed against Candida is the B-vitamin biotin. Research in Japan has indicated a fascinating way in which Candida can be deterred from altering from its relatively harmless yeast form, into its invasive and dangerous mycelial form.[17] This alteration of form is found to occur more rapidly in a medium in which there is a relative biotin deficiency. Biotin, which has also been called vitamin H, produces a number of skin conditions when known deficiency occurs in humans. These include a dermatitis which is characterized by a greyish, dry, flaky appearance. This is accompanied by a lack of appetite, nausea, lassitude and muscular pains. It is interesting that all of these symptoms are common when Candida is proliferating, and it is worth questioning whether the supposed symptoms of biotin deficiency are not at least in part the result of Candida activity brought about by that deficiency.

Egg-white contains a substance called avidin, which is capable of combining with biotin, thus neutralizing its usefulness in the body. For this reason raw egg should not be included in the anti-Candida diet (avidin is destroyed by cooking).

Biotin should be taken as a supplement, three times daily, in doses of between 350 and 500mcg in association with acidophilus (i.e. between meals).

Garlic as an Anti-Candida Agent

Garlic has been the subject of research worldwide. Russian scientists have proved the reality of its long-reputed antibacterial quality by the introduction of garlic extract into colonies of bacteria, which ceased to function within minutes. Fresh garlic juice was employed in these tests. Reports in Western medical and scientific journals confirm such claims,[18] in this case against *Salmonella typhimurium* and *Escherichia coli*, two extremely active micro-organisms. Garlic is also active against yeast and fungi. This was confirmed in recent reports showing it to be more active against human ringworm (a fungal infection) than currently used drugs.[19] *The Book of Garlic* quotes researchers as stating, 'garlic in the form of juice is a very potent anti-microbial agent, both to bacteria, and *Pathogenic yeasts*. We can thus suppose at least staphyloccocal and fungal skin and alimentary tract disease can be effectively cured by the juice of garlic.'[20]

Research at the University of Indiana suggests the value of garlic against fungal infections is very great. 'An aqueous extract of garlic bulbs inhibits growth of many aspects of zoopathogenic fungi,' the first report stated.[21]

The second concluded, 'Allicin [the active sulphur-rich compound in garlic] may provide the model system for chemotherapy of *Candida albicans* infections.'[22]

The aesthetic aspect of garlic's employment is of course a factor to consider. Whilst there are many who can happily eat whole cloves of garlic, there are others who find the taste and odour unpleasant. The recent development of a completely odourless garlic (Kyolic) is a boon to such as these. (See 'Further Information' for suppliers.)

Part of the anti-Candida campaign should include the daily intake of either fresh garlic or deodorized garlic in capsule form. The former is preferred; the latter is an acceptable compromise. Take 2-3 garlic capsules, morning and evening, after meals, or eat as much raw garlic as you can learn to enjoy. Slice it finely on cooked vegetables, or crush it on to salads, or simply eat it, clove by clove, with fish or poultry, as many Greeks do.

A further aid in the prevention of the transformation of Candida to its mycelial form is the use of olive oil.[16] This contains a substance called *oleic acid*, which also acts upon the yeast in a similar way to biotin. The recommended amount of olive oil is 6 teaspoonsful of olive oil daily, divided into three doses. This can be included in the meal or taken before or after, as desired.

Immune-System Enhancement by Supplementation
In order to strengthen the immune system it is suggested that a number of nutrients be included in the programme.

The primary nutrient in this regard is vitamin C. We have discussed this vitamin's importance in the economy of the body and its defensive T-cells. These contain a very high level of vitamin C. It has been noted that the lower the vitamin C content of these vital cells the less efficient is their performance in defending the body against intruding organisms or materials.[6, 7] Any stress factor, pollutant or infection puts demands upon the vitamin C in the body.

This is a water-soluble vitamin, and the body has no stores of it, so a constant supply is needed. Research has shown a fascinating adaptation which takes place when requirements increase because of such factors as those described above. Under normal conditions, if a person takes more vitamin C than they actually require, they are likely to develop a degree of diarrhoea. This is well known, and it is a way of assessing just how much vitamin C a person needs. If someone takes 5g daily, with no diarrhoea resulting, then they can be assumed to need that amount, at that time. If under normal conditions, however, someone develops diarrhoea after ingesting only 2g daily, it can be shown that should circumstances alter, and the need for vitamin C becomes apparent (owing to infection, stress, etc.) then that same person could increase vitamin C intake by many times the previous tolerance level, without any bowel symptoms at all. Dr Robert Cathcart has shown that if necessary the intake of vitamin C can be as high as 100g a day (never try this without supervision), with no bowel sensitivity apparent.[23] When the crisis passes, however, such doses would produce diarrhoea, as previously. Thus the body, in its wisdom, seems to be able to alter its function to meet particular requirements in this way. In order to assist a deficient immune system, such as might accompany a Candida spread, the recommended amount for this purpose (in the absence of any bowel reaction) is 1-3g daily, with food.

The effect of vitamin C on the T-cells depends of course on the T-cells being there to do their work. The thymus gland, which lies below the breastbone, can become relatively inactive, and one of the main nutrients which can enhance its production of T-cells, is the amino acid arginine.[24] A dose of 3g daily for a short period (say a month) will boost the thymus activity at the outset of the programme, when it is most needed. Note: If there is a history of herpes simplex infection, then do not take arginine supplementally, for it has also been found to enhance herpes activity (this is countered by another amino acid, lysine).[25]

Take the arginine before retiring, on an empty stomach, with water. A long-term use of arginine at these levels is not suggested, although there are no known side-effects in doses lower than 20g daily. Rough, thickened skin may develop on the elbows, for example, in doses of above 20g daily, though this will disappear when the supplementation is stopped. The reason for suggesting a time limit to the use of arginine is that the thymus may come to depend upon such nutritional supplementation, whereas it should be encouraged to return to normal activity by the total programme of Candida suppression. Therefore take the 3g daily for only the first month of this programme.

It is a further aid to the immune system to increase the intake of certain of the B-vitamins.[6] It is important to the programme that these are not derived from yeast sources.[2,9] All the B-vitamins are available in synthetic forms, and these rather than yeast-derived vitamins, are suggested in cases involving Candida. Between 20 and 50 mg of vitamin B6 (pyridoxine); between 20 and 50 mcg of vitamin B12, and the same quantity of folic acid, should be taken daily. An excellent non-yeast source B-complex capsule is available in the UK. (See 'Further Information' for supplier.)

An additional B-vitamin (B5), should also be taken to assist in the enhancement of the B-lymphocytes, especially if there is any evidence of allergic reactions, or digestive involvement. This should be taken in the form of calcium pantothenate, at a dose of 500mg daily.

The minerals zinc, selenium and magnesium are all also commonly implicated in deficient immune response conditions, [5, 6, 11] and should ideally be added to the programme. Just as in the selection of B-vitamins, it is important, in obtaining selenium, that a non-yeast source is found. This may prove difficult, but if sufficient demand is forthcoming then such problems will diminish and supply will become more plentiful. Doses required of these minerals are as follows: zinc (in the form of zinc-orotate), 50mg daily; selenium, 50mcg daily; and magnesium, 250-500mg daily. All should be taken with food.

Finally, a supply of some of the fat-soluble vitamins is called for in our effort to resuscitate the immune response. This calls for a moderate intake of vitamin E (make sure that you are buying natural vitamin E, which can be identified by the name *d*-alpha tocopherol, rather than *dl*-alpha tocopherol, which indicates a synthetic form), at a dose of around 200i.u. daily, Vitamin A in the form of beta-carotene, in a dose of around 10,000i.u. daily, and finally the oil of Evening Primrose (vitamin F), in a 500mg capsule twice daily.

Supplement List
Anti-Candida:
Lactobacillus acidophilus, 2g one to three times daily, between meals (Superdophilus or Vital Dophilus for preference).

Biotin (vitamin H) 350-500mcg with acidophilus, three times daily.

Garlic capsules (if fresh garlic is not being eaten prolifically). Three capsules, twice daily (morning and evening), after meals (Kyolic recommended – deodorized form).

Oleic acid (as virgin, first-pressing, olive oil), 2 teaspoonsful three times daily. Can be taken with meals or separately.

To Enhance Immune-System:
Vitamin C, 1g three times daily with meals.

Arginine, 3g (with water), on an empty stomach, before retiring. Take for one month only.

Vitamin B6 (pyridoxine),20-50mg daily.
Vitamin B12, 20-50mcg daily.
Folic acid, 20-50mcg daily.

} Or one vitamin B-complex capsule daily (yeast-free)

Calcium pantothenate (B5), 500mg daily (especially if allergy symptoms present).

Selenium, 50mcg daily.

Zinc, 50mg daily.

✓ *Magnesium*, 250-500mg daily.

Vitamin E (d-alpha tocopherol), 200i.u. daily.

✓ *Vitamin A* (as beta-carotene), 10,000i.u. daily.

✓ *Vitamin F* (as oil of Evening Primrose),one to two 500mg capsules daily.

Note: Ensure vitamin C is 'with bioflavonoids'; ensure that B-vitamins and selenium are not from yeast source; ensure that zinc and magnesium are orotate form (B-13 zinc, and B-13 magnesium).

It will be clear from the above that we are using the supplements in two directions at the same time.

Firstly we are using acidophilus and biotin (as well as oleic acid) as substances which directly inhibit the alteration of Candida to its dangerous fungal form, or which resist its spread. The other nutrients are employed to build up the immune function (B- and T-cells) so that the body can better cope with the invading micro-organism. This two-pronged attack requires that you take this large number of supplements at the same time. This is both moderately expensive, and off-putting. Let it be clear, however, that what is at stake is your health. For this reason there should be no hesitation in grasping this opportunity to fight off the cause of your ill health by whatever safe

methods are at hand. The methods that are being advocated
are safe. They are also effective in most cases. It can take
time to control Candida once it is rampant, and six
months should be seen as the minimum length of time to
maintain this programme.

Our next consideration is the importance of combining
the supplemental attack on Candida, and the enhancement
of the immune system, with a dietary programme which
deprives the yeast of its main sources of food.

Anti-Candida Diet

There are two major areas of consideration in the dietary
pattern necessary to reduce the spread and activity of
Candida. These are the elimination of all foods derived
from, or containing, yeasts or fungi; the second is the
reduction, as far as possible, of all carbohydrate-rich
foods, in order to deprive Candida of its favourite nourish-
ment, which as anyone who has made beer or wine will
testify, is sugar.

Foods Derived from or Containing Fungi and Yeast

The following list of foods and substances contain yeast
or yeast-like substances, and so should be avoided as
much as possible during the initial stages of dealing with
Candida infection. It is probably wise to maintain vigilance
for these foods for at least three months, after which time
a degree of relaxation can be exercised, with the proviso
that if such foods are reintroduced, and symptoms which
had become quiescent begin to become active again, a
return to a stricter mode of eating for a time is called for.
The rationale behind such avoidance is that in practice
these foods seem to aggravate a Candida-induced condition,
especially if allergic symptoms are part of the picture, as
well as if there are symptoms such as bloating and
intestinal gas.[2, 9] In a letter Dr Truss states:

If someone has no symptoms, I see no reason to have

him avoid these yeast promoting foods, although I will say that in excess, and combined with a high-carbohydrate intake [sugars, etc.], these may actually induce this condition [Candida infection] even without the stimulatory effects of antibiotics, birth control pills, cortisone, etc.

Yeast-Promoting Foods and Substances
The following foods contain yeast as an added ingredient in their preparations,[26] and are therefore undesirable, especially in the early stages of an anti-Candida programme.

Breads (non-yeasted whole wheat or corn bread is acceptable).
Cakes and cake mixes.
Biscuits and crackers.
Enriched flour.
Buns, rolls and pastries.
Anything fried in breadcrumbs (fish fingers, etc.).

The following contain yeast, or yeast-like substances, because of the nature of their manufacture, or of their own nature.

Mushrooms.
Truffles.
Soya sauce.
Buttermilk and sour cream.
Black tea.
All cheeses, including cottage cheese.
Citric acid (almost always a yeast derivative).
Citrus drinks if canned or frozen.
All dried fruits.
All fermented beverages, such as beer, spirits, wine, cider, ginger ale.
All malted products (cereals, sweets or dairy products which have been malted).

All foods containing monosodium glutamate (which is often a yeast derivative).

All vinegars, whether grape, malt, cider or anything else. These are frequently used in sauces and relishes, as well as salad dressings, sauerkraut, olives and pickled foods.

The following are either derived from yeast, or contain elements that are.

Antibiotics.

Multivitamin tablets (unless specifically stating that they are from a non-yeast source).

B-complex vitamins (unless specifically stating that they are from a non-yeast source).

Selenium (as above).

Individual B-vitamins (as above).

Dr Truss singles out some foods from this long list as the main culprits in his eyes. He states: 'It is my belief that there are several foods that are primarily to be avoided. These include all fermented drinks, as well as vinegar, mushrooms, and mouldy cheeses. I allow my patients to have cottage cheese, as well as yogurt.' He goes on further to say, 'It is rational to remove all of these foods from the diet, only if there is an indication that patients are having trouble with yeast [Candida].'[27]

In this light it should be clear that the elimination of all alcoholic beverages and vinegar (and its by-products, as listed) as well as the foregoing of the joys of blue cheeses, and the eating of mushrooms, are the major areas of alteration for some months to come, apart, that is, from the reduction in refined carbohydrates and foods rich in sugar, which we will now consider.

Sugar-Rich Foods

Sugar (sucrose) itself, in whatever guise, is to be strictly avoided during the battle to control Candida. This means white sugar, brown sugar, black sugar, and any shades in between. There is no such thing as a healthy sugar. We do not need sugar, as such, for health, and its sole claim for our attention is its taste, which it is quite easy to do without. All sugar will aid the growth and proliferation of yeast. This includes syrups, honey (yes, I'm afraid so) and other forms of sugar, such as fructose, maltose, glucose, sorbitol, etc. It includes molasses, date sugar, maple sugar and in fact all of that range of non-foods with which our real foods and beverages have been sweetened. Sweets, chocolates and all soft drinks should also be totally avoided. Honey may come as a surprise to you in this context. I myself had assumed that honey was relatively safe, in that it did not seem, to my knowledge, to become mouldy. I was corrected by Dr Truss who communicated the fact that honey does indeed contain yeast spores. He pointed out, 'Species of Zygosaccharomyces [a yeast] have been found particularly active in causing yeast spoilage of honey.' It is known that honey is indeed hygroscopic (it absorbs water) and that at a certain degree of moisture content there will be sufficient water at the surface to lower the concentration of sugars to a point that the yeasts and bacteria which might be present, can grow. Thus yeasts and other micro-organisms capable of surviving in concentrated sugar solutions (in which no yeast will grow) at a certain point in the dilution of that medium, become able to thrive. In order to prevent this from happening, honey is heated, and often has additives mixed with it, such as sodium benzoate, which inhibit the growth of fermenting yeasts. Truss and Crook both insist that honey be added to the list of banned foods during the anti-Candida campaign, and this is also my view. The length of time that this will be necessary will depend upon the speed of recovery. It should not be anticipated to be less than three months, and is more likely to be six.

The most important single dietary alteration that the

Candida sufferer can make is the removal from the diet of sugar-rich foods.

As has already been discussed, the undesirability of eating yeast-containing foods at this time removes from the scene bread, pastry, biscuits and cakes, etc. This is doubly necessary, since these are in the main undesirable because of their high carbohydrate content (unless totally wholegrain).

Any carbohydrate which has been refined beyond the simple grinding stage is undesirable. Whole wheat, or oats as employed in making porridge, or millet, or brown rice, are all highly desirable foods, rich in what are known as complex carbohydrates. These can, and indeed should (especially oats) be a part of the diet. Once these are broken down into fine flours, and are refined further, they become less desirable, and actually become food for the yeast, rather than for you.

So even in the middle stages of the programme when, hopefully, symptoms are on the wane, and you might justifiably feel that a little relaxation of the stricter aspects of the diet are allowable, please remember that refined carbohydrates are the natural food of yeast, and Candida will thank you for the delivery of such foods by a rapid expansion of its activity. As Truss puts it, 'Decreased availability of carbohydrates slows the rate of multiplication of yeast cells, and thus should reduce the amount of yeast products entering the blood stream.' The converse is true as well: the more of these foods there are in the diet, the greater will the chances be of further spread of Candida. So out of the diet goes pasta, pastry, flour products of all sorts, biscuits, cakes, buns, rolls, bread (unless any of these are made with whole grains, and without yeast or sugar).

Many foods have 'hidden sugar', in that there is sugar added in the processing or preparation. These are often foods with which sugar is not usually associated. Frozen peas, most canned foods, and many packaged and processed foods, all contain either refined flour products, or sugar, or both. For this reason, as well as for the general undesirability of many such foods from a nutritional viewpoint, these should be avoided. Not only are you actually providing the favourite foods of the yeasts within your body when you eat sugar, you are also causing a degree of metabolic and physiological mayhem.

It should be recalled that until about 100 years ago, the average annual intake of sugar in Western countries was in the region of 20lb per head. Even this was a part of the dietary pattern which included far more 'natural' vitamin- and mineral-rich foods than is currently the case. The present annual intake of sugar in the UK and USA is over 100lb per head of the population. The human body is most adaptable, but it takes more than a century to get used to such a change in nutritional intake.

Organs such as the pancreas (the source of insulin and essential protein digesting enzymes) are grossly over- worked when sugar plays a large part in the diet. The pancreas, when faced with sugar, pumps out insulin. This has the job of maintaining the proper level of sugar in the bloodstream. Insulin is also released in response to stimulant drinks, such as coffee and tea, which initially cause a release by the liver of stored sugar (as does stress). Thus a diet rich in sugar, and which contains the usual pattern of tea, coffee and alcohol (as well as cola drinks and chocolates, which also contain caffeine to stimulate this cycle) will produce a situation in which a major organ is grossly overworked. In this sort of pattern, the fluc- tuations in blood-sugar levels, boosted by dietary and liver-stored sugar, and then depressed and controlled by the pancreatic insulin, have a profound effect upon health and personality of the individual. At the same time it is noted that because of the sugar-rich diet, it is less likely that the individual will eat enough foods containing vitamins and minerals to allow him to meet the minimum standards of nutrition. Thus other systems in the body become deficient, including the immune system. This whole process may of course take years, all the while accompanied by declining well-being and an unseen rise in Candida activity. Sugar has been well described as pure, white and deadly.

It is suggested that in the first few weeks of the programme (say three weeks for safety) even fresh fruit should be avoided, because of its high content of natural fruit sugars. Even when fruit is resumed after the three-week break, it should not include the very sweet melons, which are too high in sugar for the Candida sufferer (and often contain mould).

Milk contains its own form of sugar, and this too is thought to be undesirable throughout the programme. Pasteurized milk encourages Candida.[9] The exception to this is yogurt – if it is natural and 'live', which will be clearly stated on its container. There are many 'dead' yogurts about, and a good many that have sugar added. These are quite unsuitable to the programme. Yogurt itself is helpful since it contains (when 'live') bacteria which inhibit Candida, and which assist in the repopulation of the bowel (along with acidophilus, which is often used in yogurt culture).

Other Foods to Avoid
It is best to avoid smoked meats and fish, sausages, corned beef, hot dogs and hamburgers because of the substances added to them, some of which derive from yeasts. Nuts, other than freshly cracked ones, should also be avoided, because of the degree of mould that these attract as they become rancid. Any foods which have been kept for a while, other than in a frozen state, are liable to be slightly mouldy, and these should be avoided too.

You now have a picture of the type of foods not to eat:

mainly the yeast- and fungus-related foods, as well as the refined carbohydrates, and anything containing them.

The degree of adherence to such a programme that is possible, depends upon many factors, but none less than motivation. Just how much do you want to get better, and just how much effort are you prepared to make in that quest? It is really not up to anyone but you. Certainly the taking of the supplements, as described, will go a long way towards that end. So will avoidance of yeasts and foods derived from them. But by putting the whole programme together, including the sugar-free aspect of the diet, you really give the whole system a chance to work quickly, and work well.

What you can still eat is varied and exciting. Below I have outlined a pattern of eating which is nutritious, tasty and above all 'anti-Candida' in its format.

Once you have tried to follow this type of pattern for a while, it is unlikely that you will ever really want to reintroduce most of the 'undesirables', even when Candida is back under control.

Dietary Pattern
Breakfast: It has been found that a high-fibre diet is the best suited to the resolution of the Candida problem. In Professor Jeffrey Bland's words, 'The diet should be higher than normal in fibre, using oat bran fibre to increase the absorptive surface of the faecal material and also hasten the elimination of metabolic by-products.'[16] Choose therefore from the following, for a wholesome and non-Candida-supporting breakfast. In passing, it is suggested that three meals are eaten daily, and that meals are not skipped unless you are off-colour and really have no appetite.

Choose one or more of the following for breakfast:

1. Oatmeal porridge. Add a little cinnamon and some

ground cashew nuts for additional flavour. Use no sugar or honey. Make with water, not milk.

2. Mixed seed and nut breakfast (combine sunflower, pumpkin, sesame and linseed together, with oatmeal or flaked millet). These can be eaten as they are, or soaked overnight in a little water to make a softer texture, or moistened with natural live yogurt. Add wheatgerm and freshly milled nuts if desired.

3. Alternate days: two eggs, any style except raw.

4. Bread or toast (made without yeast or sugar) and butter.

5. Brown rice kedgeree (rice and fish).

6. Wholewheat or rice and oat pancakes (no sweetening).

7. Natural live yogurt (add wheatgerm if desired).

8. After the first three weeks or so of the programme, fresh fruit can be added to the menu; for example, item 1 or 2 could be complemented by sliced banana or grated apple, or item 7 could have fresh fruit added, or fruit could be eaten as a major part of the meal, with a handful of nuts (fresh), and/or seeds (sunflower, pumpkin, etc.).

9. Fish (not smoked) or meat (not cured or salted).

10. Wholewheat, or whole rice, flakes and yogurt (ensure no sugar in cereals). The use of muesli-type breakfast mixtures is in order if they are homemade. If shop-bought they will contain dried fruit and nuts of almost certain rancidity, and frequently sugar or honey as well. By the simple mixing of oatflakes, or millet flakes, with fresh nuts or seeds, as mentioned in item 2 above, it is possible to have a high-fibre, nutritious and tasty meal.

If items 1 or 2 are eaten, then a high fibre content will be ensured, and these are suggested as the most desirable. If any of the other choices are eaten, then add a heaped teaspoonful of linseed and bran (50:50), mixed together, to the meal or swallow at the end of the meal with a little water.

Remember to chew all food, especially carbohydrates, thoroughly. There is no way in which half-chewed carbohydrates can be digested, since the enzymes present in saliva are essential to the breakdown of these foods. For this reason it is undesirable to drink with meals, as the liquid is frequently used as a moistening agent to facilitate swallowing, which reduces efficient chewing as a result. A high-fibre meal is ideal for the provision of the type of food needed for the anti-Candida programme. It also ensures a steady release of natural sugars into the bloodstream, rather than the rapid rise produced by most refined sugar-rich foods. This helps to keep blood-sugar levels even, and avoids ups and downs in available energy (and mood) which can be a major cause of the craving for a quick 'sugar fix'.

Drinks at breakfast time should consist of either green tea, china tea, herb tea (such as Rooibos or camomile), all unsweetened, or a mineral water, such as Perrier.

Main Meals
There should be no great problem in eating quite splendid food, during the strict avoidance period of the dietary programme. One area of contention exists in the choice of animal proteins. It is important to realize that most commercial meat and poultry now contains residues of antibiotics and hormonal substances, which are fed to the animals in the process of rearing them for market. This means that regular eating of beef, pork or chicken, unless it is from a source known to avoid such methods, is a potential danger to the success of the whole programme

(and a health hazard at all times). Indeed it is not improbable that this very factor is a major, if as yet unrecognized, element in the whole Candida scenario. Whilst the use of antibiotics and steroids in medication can be relatively easily remembered and identified in the medical history, it is impossible to know just how much of these same substances are entering people on a daily basis through their food.

For this reason it is suggested that efforts be made to track down non-steroid-fed meat and poultry, in which antibiotics have not been employed. In major cities this is probably possible. Such shops as 'Wholefood' in Paddington Street, London, will guarantee such supplies. In California there is a chain of supermarkets ('Mrs Gooch's Ranch Markets') which provide a complete range of meats and poultry, guaranteed free of all contamination. Lamb and mutton is less likely to be affected by this sort of additive, as is rabbit and any other game meat, or poultry. Fish is safe, apart from other sources of pollution, which do not concern Candida directly. For the duration of the diet, therefore, it is suggested that unless the source of meat or poultry can be certainly identified as free of hormones or antibiotics, meat should be limited to game, rabbit (unless 'farmed'), mutton or lamb. Fish of course can be eaten regularly as well.

Ideally, in order to maintain the high-fibre type of meal that is so desirable when Candida is active, the two main meals of the day should include as wide a variety of fresh vegetables as is possible. These should be eaten both raw and cooked, and an excellent pattern to adopt is as follows. One of the main meals (say lunch) each day, is a source of protein such as fish, poultry, lamb, egg or fresh nuts, together with as large a mixed salad as imagination can conjure and appetite can cope with. The other main meal should also contain protein, in addition to cooked vegetables. The source of protein at each meal does not of

course have to be based on animals. The combining of a
cereal and a pulse (say brown rice and lentils, or millet and
chick-peas) at the same meal, ensures that adequate
protein is available to the body.

What is essential is that adequate protein be eaten
daily, whether from a 'safe' animal source, or from the
judicious mixing of complementary vegetable proteins.
What is adequate for one person is not necessarily so for
another. For example, people of oriental origin require,
for good health, less protein than people of northern
European stock. The difference lies in the efficiency with
which the orientals digest and absorb what they do eat in
the protein line. Thus 50g a day of first-class protein is
adequate for an oriental, and 75g (or more depending
upon activity, etc.) may be required by a European.[5]

Since natural live yogurt (a source of protein) is going
to play a part in the diet, it is unlikely that the eating of
protein at both of the main meals, in addition to this, is
necessary. It should be possible to have, for example, a
mixed salad, together with a jacket potato or savoury rice
dish, and additional nuts and seeds, for one meal, whilst
having a 'safe' animal protein and a variety of cooked
vegetables at the other. In any case the tastes and
preferences of individuals will differ markedly, and the
variations that are available as to what to eat are so great
that no more than broad guidelines can be given.
The essentials are to ensure the following:

- Avoid all yeast-based, or yeast-containing, foods.
- Avoid all sugar and refined cereal products, and foods
  containing them.
- Avoid all foods and drinks based upon fermentation.
- Avoid meats containing residues of antibiotics and
  steroids.
- Do eat three meals daily.
- Do ensure adequate protein intake.

- Do ensure that a high dietary fibre content is maintained.
- Avoid fruit for the first three or four weeks of the programme.

Once symptoms begin to abate, and you find that you would like to increase the range of foods slightly, it is of course permissible to experiment a bit. This should not be before the end of the second month on the programme, and then only if there has been a marked improvement. If you then introduce one food which has been on the 'no-go' list, observe the consequences carefully. If these are non-existent, you might extend your experiment to another food after a week or so. If symptoms return, go back to basic avoidance, as specified above, until they calm down again. I am not saying they you *must* experiment in this way, only that if you must, or if you feel constrained by the limitation imposed by the programme, then at least do it carefully, with the knowledge that it might (only might) upset things. If it does, it just means being patient for a little longer. There are many excellent books available which explain the principles of rotation diets which can help in formulating a strategy for eating certain foods only periodically in a systematic way.[28] It is not suggested that the reintroduction of sugar-containing foods be started at this stage, other than in the very minimal sense or perhaps introducing something such as pasta or honey.

Other Essential Information Regarding Food
Moulds are present on most fruits and vegetables, and these should be kept well washed and eaten fresh, for obviously the longer they are kept, the more the mould development will be encouraged.

Yeasts also grow on grains of all sorts, and the fresher these are the better. A good many people with Candida problems are allergic to grains. This allergy may well diminish during the programme of Candida control, and a little experimentation is in order after two or three months if symptoms generally have declined. A reminder is called for regarding nuts. Peanuts and pistachios, in particular, are subject to mould development (in the case of peanuts this is a highly toxic, potentially cancer-causing agent). All nuts, unless freshly opened by you, will contain some degree of mould, and certainly a degree of rancidity of the natural oils. Eat current season nuts, freshly opened by yourself, or else avoid them.

Apart from a little butter, and natural live yogurt, it is suggested that all milk products be avoided (Dr Truss does allow cottage cheese).

If you are forced to eat at a restaurant, or if friends invite you for a meal, then make sure that you stick to basics. Avoid sauces and gravy; avoid desserts; avoid stuffing, or any obvious undesirables, such as mushrooms. A meat, poultry or fish dish, with salad or vegetables, is the safest bet, and stick to water instead of wine.

What about sugar substitutes for those who cannot keep away from sweet things? These are open to question, as far as long-term safety is concerned, but in small amounts, for the duration of the programme (at least six months) they at least do not encourage Candida. Aspartame and saccharin fall into this category, but not fructose, corn syrup or any other sugar-rich substitute for the real thing.

Remember that all commercial breakfast foods, such as cornflakes, are undesirable. They are processed, and most contain yeast and/or sugar products.

Water from the tap should be filtered before drinking if possible. There are many inexpensive water filters available, and this will remove a variety of organic substances which otherwise find their way into food, or directly into you. Most bottled water is acceptable, but ensure this is not carbonated if you have problems with bloating and gas. As for coffee and tea, this is a sticking point for many. They are undesirable, not only as sources of mould, but because they stimulate sugar release from the liver, and consequently (a) pancreatic activity, which exhausts this vital organ further, and (b) the feeding of Candida by this sugar. There are other good reasons for not using tea, as it reduces the efficiency of both protein and iron absorption by the body; and coffee is suspected of involvement in certain forms of cancer. Herb teas are often better, and some have been found to help in the control of Candida, and related problems (Rooibos, a South African tea, used as a tea substitute, and by allergic subjects) and taheebo (helpful in catarrhal problems), etc., are worth trying, if you can find them (try a health food store).

The steaming of vegetables is the best way to help to retain the vital minerals so often destroyed and lost in boiling. Dressing a salad with lemon juice, olive oil and a little natural yogurt can replace the vinegar or other dressings not compatible with the programme. As the programme produces its results, and symptoms become tolerable, or disappear, so can a limited quantity of foods based on or containing mould or yeast be reintroduced. Wine, or real ale, in limited amounts, or tea, etc., may be taken occasionally. However, the need for vigilance must continue, because it is not the aim of the programme to remove Candida from the scene altogether, and nor would this be possible. Even if the problem is attacked vigorously, with the use of antifungal drugs as well as the programme outlined above, the yeast will remain in the body.

The long-term answer, after initially controlling the yeast by these means, is to maintain a high level of immune function, by respect for what the diet should contain, in terms of nutrient value, as well as avoidance in the main of those factors which you now know can reduce its optimum ability to defend you. This does not mean that the programme is a life-sentence. It is hoped that after a while you will come to regard sweet tastes as unpleasant, and no longer crave, or even enjoy sweet foods. It is also to be hoped that your new sense of well-being will help to motivate you towards following the pattern of eating suggested more or less permanently, because you will actually enjoy it, as well as because it is good for you.

Other Factors

It is important not only to avoid foods and beverages containing fungal or yeast substances, but also to avoid inhaling these organisms or their spores. This is the reason for keeping well away from damp, dank places and for dealing with the presence of any mould and wet or dry rot that might be present in your environment.If there is any danger of damp in rooms, cupboards, cellars or lofts, do something positive about dealing with this, or, if absolutely necessary, move to a new, dry place of residence. *Your home might be making you ill.*

This advice is especially applicable to anyone who notices a worsening of symptoms in weather that is damp or muggy, or who is obviously affected by contact with mouldy or dank environments.

The availability to you of full-spectrum light is another important element which can improve immune and general function.[29] It is known that the eyes contain photo-receptors which carry impulses directly to the pituitary gland, which lies in the head. This is the 'master' gland of the body and is vital for normal health and function. If light is denied the eyes (not artificial light, but the full spectrum from the sun) then demonstrable imbalances occur in the hormonal system as a direct result. Behavioural and physical symptoms can occur in consequence. The immune system is affected, and this is the reason for our interest. The advice to all who wear glasses, or who spend most of their days indoors behind glass, is that they should get outside for at least half an hour a day, with nothing between natural light and their eyes. If going out is not possible, then spend the time by an open window, without glasses or contact lenses. In a polluted city the light getting through is distorted to a degree, and so more exposure is required. This does not mean looking at the sun, even on an overcast day; just being outdoors is enough if the eyes are not shielded.

There are now available full-spectrum fluorescent lighting units (address in Further Information). It has been found that health and productivity improve dramatically when such lighting is introduced into the workplace. As one of the additional supports for the immune system, the implementation of access to unpolluted, unfiltered, pure light is a positive step.

The immune system also benefits from adequate exercise. This means trying to apply the ideals set out in Dr Kenneth Cooper's book *Aerobics*.[30] As least every other day there should be a form of physical exercise sufficient to stimulate the circulation and respiration. A brisk walk of one or two miles is the safest and easiest form of exercise that can produce such results. The book mentioned should be read, and its graded advice followed. Its beauty lies in the way in which it is made applicable to anyone, at any stage of fitness, or otherwise, so that the reader can gradually lift himself to his own level of optimum fitness in slow stages.

The avoidance of stress and anxiety is a fundamental need, as is the requirement we all have for what has been called TLC (tender loving care). These ingredients for a healthy life have been well described in many popular and readily available books. The requirement of the immune system for such inputs should encourage the study of relaxation and meditation and general stress-reducing methods. I have outlined a programme of stress reduction in my book on the subject,[31] and this should be helpful in both assessing and dealing with those stress factors which affect life. In considering the overall importance of the immune system, it is worth commenting upon an area of medical research which tends to be ignored, because of its unpopular message. There is abundant proof that women who are promiscuous, or who have relations with a large number of men, are more prone to cancer of the womb than those who have relations with only one or a few partners.[5] Early sexual experience is also shown to pre-dispose the individual towards diseases which should be prevented by an intact immune system.

AIDS is more common among homosexuals who have multiple partners, rather than those who have steady relationships with a single partner. It would seem therefore that what is happening is that in close physical contact of a sexual nature there is a role for the immune system. It is assumed that if this is called upon to cope with antigens from a wide variety of different sources (remember that sperm is a foreign protein to the body) then it could well be a factor in depleting the immune response of an individual (along with a great number of other factors).

This viewpoint has been expressed in numerous medical journals since the AIDS epidemic began.[32] It points to a necessary return to relative fidelity, in sexual terms, as being desirable for anyone who wishes to maintain an intact immune system. This does not mean that celibacy is called for, but that frequent changes in sexual partners are to be avoided. This is desirable both in heterosexual and homosexual relationships, at the very least during the carrying out of the programme against Candida.

We will briefly consider other methods by which some practitioners attempt to control Candida.

Note: It should be clear from the earlier discussions that there should be no intake of antibiotics, steroids or the contraceptive pill during the course of the anti-Candida programme unless absolutely vital.

6.

ADDITIONAL METHODS OF CANDIDA CONTROL

Nystatin
The treatment of fungal infection, such as Candida, by drug methods, involves the use of antifungal antibiotics, such as nystatin. This is active against a wide range of yeasts, and yeast-like fungi, including Candida. This drug comes in a variety of forms: as a liquid, for use in the mouth; as tablets, for use in treating Candida in the intestinal tract; as suppositories, for use in the vagina; and as creams, ointments and powders, for the treatment of surface areas, nails, etc.

Nystatin is lethal to yeast cells on contact. Getting them into contact is not always easy, especially if the area involved is deep in the bowel. The nystatin, passing through, will kill surface yeasts, but any that are imbedded deeper into the wall of the intestine will remain untouched. There is poor absorption of nystatin, so little reaches the bloodstream.

There is general consensus that nystatin is well tolerated, and causes few side-effects.[2, 9] The major reason for not opting for its use is that it deals only with the short-term situation. If a condition such as Candida has become so widespread as to cause a problem, then it is vital that the immune system and bowel flora which should be controlling the situation are revitalized. Reliance on nystatin will leave the immune system in the same state, except that there will, over a period, be fewer yeast by-products entering the bloodstream to challenge the immune system. This, it is thought (Truss, Crook, etc.), allows the immune system to revive gradually. There is certainly no objection to nystatin being employed if the condition is severe enough to warrant it, but this should only be done in combination with the sort of programme outlined in the previous chapters. Otherwise there will be but short-term gains and the condition will recur. It is important to realize that nystatin is itself derived from a mould source and can cause allergic symptoms in sensitive individuals. Some patients become dependent on nystatin and find difficulty in being weaned from it.

The dosage of nystatin (available in UK as 'Nystan', manufactured by E. R. Squibb & Sons) is usually around 2 million units daily (4 tablets of half a million units each), but double this dosage is relatively safe. Side-effects are limited to nausea, vomiting and diarrhoea, which occur only with very high doses (over 4 million units daily).

The above information should not be taken as an explicit recommendation for the use of nystatin. The major recommendations given in this book regarding the control of Candida by natural rather than drug methods are effective in the majority of cases. Taking nystatin does not necessarily shorten the process of control, and indeed may result in the individual relying on the drug and thus allowing the supporting anti-Candida programme to lapse.

By relying on the dietary and supplementation programme it is not only possible to control Candida, but to improve general well-being dramatically. This is something no drug can achieve, however few side-effects it produces.

Copper Aspirinate

Bland has discussed the usefulness in the treatment of Candida of a combination of the mineral copper with aspirin, in the form of a copper aspirinate compound. This, he points out,[16] provides, in one tablet, 10mg of copper daily and 330mg of aspirin. This apparently reduces the symptoms of Candida infection associated with intestinal irritation and inflammation. He describes the research of Dr J. Sorenson who has called this preparation 'one of the most powerful anti-flammatory substances studied to date'.[33] It has both an anti-flammatory and an anti-fungal role to play according to this research.

As far as the use of copper aspirinate in the anti-Candida programme is concerned, it must be clear that while being of possible short-term use, it does not comply with the description 'natural', in that this is clearly a pharmaceutical (drug) effect that is being aimed at, rather than the bolstering of the defence mechanism, or a biological attack upon Candida, such as is foreseen in using acidophilus. This does not mean that copper aspirinate should not be used, only that it does not form part of the programme recommended in this book. Its limited availability is another factor not making it at least an alternative in the opening phases of the programme. Bland suggests its use, especially in cases in which intestinal factors play a large part in the symptom picture, for the first two to three weeks of the programme.

Caprystatin

The antifungal activity of certain fatty acids has been demonstrated by investigators such as Neuhauser[40] who has shown dilute (0.01) caprylic acid (coconut extract) to destroy Candida effectively. He has successfully treated patients with severe intestinal Candida by using caprylic acid in a form which allows a timed release as it passes through the bowel. If not in such a form the caprylic acid is ineffective, being absorbed in the upper intestinal region. Caprylic acid mimics the fatty acids produced by normal bowel flora, which are a major factor in the body's control over Candida. As yet available only via its US manufacturers (see 'Further Information' for address) public demand for this would rapidly result in UK availability.

Colonics and Enemas

Colonic irrigation involves the administration of water into the bowel, sometimes combined with other substances, in order to clear debris from the region and to influence its health. Useful in this respect are garlic extract, oxygen and acidophilus (or as Crook suggests, nystatin). By making repeated applications of water, coupled with one of these additives, there is every chance of greatly influencing the condition of the bowel. Enemas are less effective, since they penetrate only a short distance, unlike the colonic which can pass water the length of the large bowel. The technique requires expert skills, and its use in Candida problems would require additional knowledge. In principle, however, such treatment is recommended, at least in the early stages of the programme. There is no reason why acidophilus should not itself be adminstered in this way rather than orally alone, to assist in the repopulation of the bowel and control of Candida.

Desensitization

Carefully controlled doses of Candida extract may be injected into the individual in the hope that this will produce a response on the part of the immune system. Antibodies thus produced by white blood cells are useful in assisting the defence against antigens entering the system because of the yeast. The use of yeast extracts as a 'vaccine' of this sort also appears to assist general immune function, by helping to balance or regulate aspects of the system relating to 'helper' and 'suppressor' cells, as discussed earlier (see Chapter 2).

The whole exercise is complicated in the extreme, because whilst *Candida albicans* is a strain of yeast which is clearly identifiable, it contains within its make-up, a large number of variables. Thus the Candida which is growing in one person is not exactly the same as that growing in another. This biological individuality applies to yeasts just as much as to every other living creature, including people. Thus the same extract of Candida, injected into two people, will not produce the same response. Not only is the yeast likely to prove different from that to which the individual is normally exposed, but his/her individuality, superimposed upon that fact, makes for a process of trial and error, in achieving a response which is going to help the individual's immune system to fight the particular strain of Candida present in his system. Hereditary factors may largely be responsible for the differences in response of individuals to such treatment, and this requires that whoever is employing anti-Candida desensitization treatment be expert in the field and be able to cope with the complex variables.

Even should such expertise be available, this approach, with all its possible pitfalls in terms of variable reactions, can at best deal with just one aspect of the problem. It may assist in bolstering the immune system against the by-products of Candida's infestation. This is especially desirable for those people who are suffering from the type of allergy symptoms mentioned earlier. But it will do little for the local symptoms currently active in the bowel or reproductive system. Only those aspects of Candida's harmful effects which are mediated by the bloodstream will be helped. Valuable as this may be, it would leave much of the underlying condition the same, and would still necessitate that the programme of anti-Candida diet and supplements be implemented, in order to control its spread and deny it its nutrients.

Truss points out that the use of this type of 'vaccination' programme is contra-indicated in patients suffering from what are called auto-immune conditions. These include rheumatoid arthritis. Stimulation of the immune response in someone who is being attacked by his own immune system would lead to aggravation of this condition. Truss has written:

> I obtain yeast from supply houses that have been made aware of the necessity of bio-assaying each new batch on humans. Prior to their being informed of this fact, they were putting out a number of batches that would not give a positive skin test on known reactors. The preparation as I order it, is simply Candida albicans 1:10.[34]

This indicates one more pitfall in this method: it is vital that the Candida extract used is actually active, and that this has been proven in each batch produced, otherwise the pitfalls described above are compound.

These two major anti-Candida methods are the major forms of treatment recommended by both Dr Truss and Dr Crook. They do of course strongly advocate the dietary approach, especially in the prevention of Candida spreading, as well as being supportive of these treatments.

The natural approach to the control of Candida has been outlined in previous chapters, and the reader must choose for himself the method that appeals the most.

The following case histories will give an indication of the way in which this 'natural' approach works.

7.

CASE HISTORIES

Mr E. M., age 36
This young man, employed as a local government officer,
consulted me in 1982 after seven years, during which his
health had declined dramatically. His major symptoms
(and there were others) included bloating of the abdomen,
accompanied by nausea and flatulence, heartburn and
indigestion. Constipation had become chronic. There
was a tendency to light-headedness and dizziness. There
were periodic attacks of shivering, followed by high
temperature, which incapacitated him.

The onset of the condition, previous to which his
health was unremarkable, came after an attack of gastro-
enteritis whilst on holiday. Treatment had, naturally
enough, been with a broad-spectrum antibiotic. In his
own words,

> For the eighteen months following [the gastro-enteritis]
> I suffered all the symptoms daily, which were so severe
> it resulted in my being unable to attend work for six
> months continuously, and the remaining twelve months
> I attended only with massive support from my colleagues,
> who shared my work load, and understanding superiors

who allowed me to go home, or rest, when the attacks were extremely severe.

There had been a gradual improvement over the following years until some twelve months prior to my seeing him, when, after an acute attack, he was left with all the symptoms described above. At that time he wrote, 'At present I am struggling to cope with each day as it comes, and deal with this extremely debilitating and distressing illness as best I can.'

In these intervening years between the onset of his illness and consulting me, he had been seen by numerous medical practitioners. An endoscopy (at Charing Cross Hospital) showed no disease of the bowel. He was checked for what is called a malabsorption problem, and again no abnormality was discerned. He went to the Royal Homoeopathic Hospital on two occasions, and consulted a herbalist, an osteopath and a medical specialist in allergies (a clinical ecologist). He had been placed on a rotation diet, which helped him to avoid repetitive contact with suspected food families, but which had little effect on his condition.

At the time I first saw him his diet was as follows. Breakfast: *Bacon* and tomato or *sausages*. *Rice cakes* and *marmalade*. Decaffeinated *coffee* and *fruit juice* (not freshly made). Mid-morning he had fresh fruit. Lunch was a salad and baked potato plus *ham* or cottage cheese. The evening meal was either *chicken* or *pork* or *sausages* or fish and vegetables. He had *rice cakes* and a hot *milk* drink before retiring. I have italicized those aspects of his eating pattern which are contra-indicated in an anti-Candida diet.

He appeared exhausted, but was a bright and intelligent patient who I felt would co-operate actively in any programme designed to assist recovery.

After tests including cytoxic tests to elicit specific

foods to which he might be reacting as well as hair analysis (low in chromium, iron, manganese and selenium), he was prescribed the following:

1. An anti-yeast, anti-fungus pattern of eating, low in carbohydrates.
2. Supplements of vitamins A, E, B1, B2, B3, B6, calcium pantothenate (B5), calcium, magnesium and manganese. Vitamin C was also added. The vitamin A was in emulsified form for easy absorption.
3. The pattern of eating was to include a seed and yogurt breakfast, a salad lunch and an evening meal of 'safe' protein with vegetables.

At this time the knowledge regarding biotin and acidophilus was not current, and the above programme, which the reader will recognize as a modified version of that given in earlier chapters, had a remarkable effect. Improvement began soon after the institution of the programme. Two months later biotin and acidophilus were introduced. When seen six months after the first visit, the report was of at least a 50 per cent improvement in all symptoms; there were still some days of exhaustion, but overall an upwards trend in the health spectrum was noted, after seven years of decline. Confirmation of the involvement of Candida came with an attempt early in the programme to introduce an organic iron supplement, in a liquid yeast-based form. This was met with an immediate return of constipation, which had more or less resolved itself. A check-up six months later found a continued improvement, with lapses in the diet producing confirmatory flare-ups. There is no reason to doubt that the condition will be kept under control, and that the health of the patient will continue to improve. A letter just eighteen months after the start of the programme states, 'Please accept apologies for delay in contacting you. It is an indication of the progress we have made that I am well enough not to have

to adhere so strictly. I am very much better overall.'
(Letter dated 8 November 1984.)

Mrs E. V., age 50

This patient consulted me with a history of extreme
itching and inflammation of the skin of the neck and
scalp, of one year's duration. She had an earlier history of
acne, which was treated by antibiotic therapy (unsuccess-
fully). She suffered from flatulence and had a history of
colitis and a 'delicate' digestive system. She had consulted
a herbalist, with little result, and a hypnotist who taught
her relaxation and helped her to stop scratching the area.
The condition remained as before. At the time of the
consultation I was not yet aware of the work of Dr Truss
on Candida and my approach was to use a nutrient
supplementation, based on her general clinical picture, a
nutritional questionnaire, a hair analysis and her current
symptoms. Her dietary pattern was excellent (which,
since this turned out to be a Candida problem, had
probably saved her from far wider infestation).

She was placed on the following supplements, each
taken daily: emulsified vitamin A, 60,000i.u.; zinc orotate,
200mg; calcium and magnesium orotates, 1g each;
chromium orotate 10mg, and selenium 50mcg; as well as
oil of Evening Primrose (vitamin F), 1g. I also suggested
she take yeast tablets as a source of vitamin B. At this
point she wrote to me (she lived a considerable distance
from my practice) saying 'I am following your suggestions
carefully, except for the brewer's yeast. Over the years I
have tried a number of times to take it, but it creates gas
and is most unpleasant.'

This set off alarm bells, for I had just read the first of Dr
Truss's articles that week. I immediately revised the
pattern of eating, which, whilst good under usual conditions,
contained substances derived from yeast, and of course a
certain amount of 'yeast food' such as honey and muesli

bars. The patient cancelled her following appointment with the comment that, as her symptoms had disappeared, she felt the journey unnecessary. I quite agreed. A year later she remained symptom-free, including both skin and bowel condition.

Mrs D. B., age 31

I was consulted by this lady, a computer-programmer, with the following list of complaints.

Eyes bloodshot and irritating, for the past nine months. Odd aches, in joints and muscles. Fingers slightly swollen. Puffiness under eyes (and sometimes above) after sleep. Ten years since the onset of this she had had cosmetic surgery and diuretics, to no avail. She had been on a macrobiotic diet as well, with no improvement.
Periods were erratic and painful. Breasts swelled and became sensitive at this time.
She felt unnaturally tired a good deal of the time.
There was a history in the family of bronchial problems and depression, from which she too suffered.

Her current diet was:

Breakfast: shop-bought *muesli with added sugar* plus *milk* or apple juice (once a week she had eggs and *bacon* and *sausage* for breakfast).

Lunch: A cooked vegetarian savoury or *sandwiches*.

Evening meal: Fish and rice, occasional meat.

During the day she had the odd *sweet* and had three cups of *tea*, plus *sugar* and *biscuits*.

She had noticed a progressive inablity to cope with alcohol. Her diet was reformed to remove the sugars and milk, and to increase complex carbohydrates. She was prescribed (after appropriate tests) vitamin B complex, kelp, oil of Evening Primrose, vitamin B2, glutamic acid (an amino acid), and the minerals chromium, iron, manganese and selenium. Also prescribed were biotin and acidophilus, after meals. Within two months she reported that her period had been on time for the first time in years, there had been a less overall tendency to swell (eyes or breasts), and she was able to cope with alcohol. (It was in fact proscribed from her diet, which raises the problem of patients complying with instructions – a major headache for practitioners.) Three months later her condition was vastly improved, and her tiredness, bloodshot eyes, aches in muscles and joints, had all diminished to a point where they no longer bothered her. A year later she was symptom-free.

Miss G. H., aged 29

The tragic progression of ill health in this case is a clear indictment of the failure of many health professionals to recognize Candida when it is staring them in the face.

Before consulting me, the lady in question wrote to me as follows:

> I have been suffering from Pelvic Inflammatory Disease (PID) for almost two years now. The problem started when I began to experience lower abdominal pain and feel generally unwell. I was, at the time, using the contraceptive IUD, which I had removed, believing this to be the cause of the pain. [Prior to this, it turned out, the young lady had been using the contraceptive pill, and had a history of recurrent thrush.] However, this [removal of the coil] had no effect and the pain became worse. Unfortunately my GP did not diagnose PID, and I therefore received no treatment in the early stages of the disease. Eventually I went to hospital, where the gynaecologist diagnosed PID through a laparoscopy. At that time there was some damage to

the fallopian tubes and adhesions in the pelvic area. I was put on to antibiotics, and for a time the condition seemed to improve. After a short time, however, I began to experience further attacks, and had to take larger doses of antibiotics regularly, and strong pain-killers for much of the time. At times the pain was incredibly intense. In January 1983 I was admitted to a Women's Hospital in London for another laparoscopy. They found that both fallopian tubes were blocked, and it sounded as though damage/adhesions in the pelvic area had progressed. Despite this I was told that the pain I was complaining of was psychological, and though they would be prepared to do tube reconstruction, for fertility purposes, there was nothing more they could do for me.

I visited a consultant, in Harley Street, in February 1983, who said that my symptoms and pain were classic PID, but there was nothing he could do to help. . .

My menstrual cycle had now gone from four to six weeks. Apart from the pain, other symptoms were active nausea, stomach upset, dizziness, slightly raised temperature. I also became very depressed. In July 1983 I had surgery after consulting a leading gynae-cologist at Hammersmith Hospital. This consisted of removal of left fallopian tube and reconstruction of the right; separation of adhesions to tubes, ovaries and uterus through microsurgery; presacral neurotomy (removal of nerve to uterus); steroid treatment to prevent regrowth of adhesions.

After this all was well until early November 1983, when symptoms began again. Although pain was not as severe, tests showed the infection was active again. I was put on heavy doses of antibiotics. It did not clear up, and I am now in my sixth week of antibiotics. The consultant told me that there was nothing more they can do surgically, and that I may have the condition for the rest of my life, and must learn to live with it. I have a very positive attitude towards getting better, and find it very difficult to believe that there is nothing else I can do to beat this disease, or at least fight it more effectively.

The patient's history indicated that she had commenced on this sad slide to ill health at the age of 12, when cystitis was first apparent, after which she soon began a thirteen-year history of vaginal thrush.

In late January of 1984, this patient was placed on the programme as outlined in earlier chapters: high fibre, low refined carbohydrate; no fungal foods; and supplements of biotin, acidophilus, olive oil, zinc, vitamin F and garlic. Two months later she reported that she was feeling quite a lot better, apart from a couple of bad spells from which she recovered more quickly than usual.

A letter dated 10 January 1985 reads as follows, 'I have been feeling considerably better. The pain problem is now limited to a few days a month (around period time). After my last laparoscopy the consultant said that it was the best result from that type of operation that he'd ever had. My remaining fallopian tube was tested and is clear, so I am a lot happier in myself'. This is a clear and dramatic example of the tragedy that occurs when Candida becomes active in a young body, and of the effectiveness of the programme outlined in this book.

Miss S. R., age 35

This young actress suffered from a continuous form of facial acne, which was both unsightly and a disadvantage in her work, as well as being psychologically upsetting. This condition had been present since the age of 14. Her past history was unremarkable, apart from a highly stressed lifestyle, a surgical intervention (cryo-surgery) to deal with a cervical erosion, and a tendency not to ovulate regularly. When under stress in the past, the skin erupted into very large pustules. By following the anti-Candida programme (as outlined in earlier chapters) her skin was normal and she was ovulating regularly, after just three months. This has been maintained for the past year.

Candida is possibly the least understood, most widespread cause of ill health currently in our midst. Precisely because it is known to be everywhere, it is largely ignored, and not even considered, when diagnosis of conditions such as that of the young lady with PID is sought. The cases quoted by Dr Truss, which include similar pictures to those described above, as well as individuals who were diagnosed as schizophrenic, manic depressives, and as having multiple sclerosis, deserve to be emphasized. All of these were restored to normality with the application of the sort of nutritional programme we have been considering, together with anti-yeast drug treatment.

A wider awareness of this diagnosis as a possibility would perhaps lead to a marked reduction in human suffering. This is not just a minor health irritant. It can destroy the physical and mental cohesion of the individual in a very short space of time. Prevention is by the same means as those described for treatment. The knowledge that we now have as to what makes Candida spread is easy to understand and easily put into practical use.

Self-help is always necessary, and until the profession of medicine becomes aware of the import of this knowledge it is vital. Past experience in this regard is not comforting. It can take 50 years, or more, for the penetration of an idea such as this to permeate the profession as a whole. Let us hope that with modern communication, and the help of the media, this will be speeded up in the case of Candida. The name of Dr C. Orion Truss, of Birmingham, Alabama, will eventually become well known throughout medicine. He is deserving of the gratitude of us all for his research into *Candida albicans* and its role as a cause of so much ill health.

FURTHER INFORMATION

Supplement Supplies
Supplements can be obtained from health food stores, or from the following suppliers:

Superdophilus available from G & G Supplies, 51 Railway Approach, East Grinstead, West Sussex. Tel. 0342-23016.

Vital Dophilus available from York Medical Supplies, 4 Museum St, York. Tel. 0904-52378.

Yeast-free B-complex available from Bio-Health Ltd, 13 Oakdale Rd, London SW16. Tel. 01-769-7975.

Caprystatin available from Arteria, 1061-B Shary Circle, Concord, California, 94518

Cantassium Co., 225 Putney Bridge Rd, London SW15 (source of minerals in orotate form, as well as biotin).

Lamberts, P.O. Box 1, Tunbridge Wells, Kent (source of supplements, as above but not orotates).

Natren Inc., 12142 Huston Street, North Hollywood, California 91607. USA (source of Megadophilus).

Four Seasons Natural Products, 52 Colegate, Norwich (source of Kyolic garlic capsules).

Full-spectrum lighting is available from Paul Temple Lighting, Holloway Lane, Harmondsworth, West Drayton, Middx.

Recommended Reading

C. Orion Truss M.D., *The Missing Diagnosis*, obtainable from author, P.O. Box 26508, Birmingham, Alabama 35226, USA.

William G. Crook M.D., *The Yeast Connection*, obtainable from author, P.O. Box 3494, Jackson, Tennessee 38301, USA.

Jeffrey Bland, *Your Personal Health Programme*, Thorsons.

Dr Michael Colgan, *Your Personal Vitamin Profile*, Blond & Briggs.

Journal of Alternative Medicine, obtainable from 30 Station Approach, West Byfleet, Surrey.

REFERENCES

1. Roger Williams, *Biochemical Individuality* (University of Texas Press, 1979).
2. C. Orion Truss M.D., *Missing Diagnosis* (see Further Information for address).
3. Jay Stein (ed.), *Internal Medicine* (Little Brown, 1983).
4. R. Williams and G. Deason, *Proceedings of National Academy of Sciences* (USA, 57, p.1638, 1968).
5. J. Bland (ed.), *Medical Application of Clinical Nutrition* (Keats, 1983).
6. Jeffrey Bland Ph.D., *Nutraerobics* (Harper & Row, 1983).
7. Dr Michael Colgan, *Your Personal Vitamin Profile* (Blond & Briggs, 1983).
8. Roger Williams Ph.D., *Nutrition against Disease* (Bantam, 1981).
9. W. M. Crook M.D., *The Yeast Connection* (Professional Books).
10. *Journal of Orthomolecular Psychiatry*, Vol. 9, No. 4 (1980), pp.287-301.
11. W. Philpott and D. Kalita, *Brain Allergies* (Keats, 1980).
12. Dr W. Hemmings, *Food Antigens in the Gut* (Lancaster Press, London, 1980).
13. K. Shahani and A. Ayeno, 'Role of dietary lactobacilli in gastrointestinal microecology', in *American Journal of Clinical Nutrition* Vol. 33 (Nov. 1980), pp.2448-57.
14. M. Speck, 'Contributions of micro-organisms to foods and nutrition', in *Nutrition News* Vol. 38, No. 4 (1975) p.13.
15. G. Reddy *et al.*, 'Natural Antibiotic activity of *Lactobacillus acidophilus* and *bulgaricus*', in *Cultured Dairy Products Journal* Vol. 18, No. 2 (1983), p.15.

16. Dr Jeffrey Bland Ph.D., 'Candida Albicans — An Alternative Therapy for an Unexpected Problem', in *Journal of Alternative Medicine*, July 1983, pp.18-19.
17. *Medical Science Proceedings* (Yamaguchi, 1982).
18. *Applied Microbiology* June 1969; Lloyd Harris, *The Book of Garlic* (Aris Books, 1979).
19. *Medical Journal of Australia* Vol. 1, No. 60 (1982).
20. Tyarcke and Gos, 'Inhibitory Action of Garlic on Growth and Respiration of Micro-organisms' (1979).
21. *Mycologia* Vol. LXVII, No. 4 (1975).
22. *Mycologia* Vol. LXIX, No. 4 (1977).
23. Robert Cathcart M.D., 'Vitamin C-Titrating to Bowel Tolerance', *Medical Hypothesis* 7: 1359-76 (1981).
24. *American Journal of Clinical Nutrition* Vol. 37, No. 5, (1983), pp.786.
25. *Dermatolgia* No. 156, (1978), pp.257-67.
26. Brown and Binkley, *Yeast: A Brief Description of Common Sources* (1980).
27. Personal Communication to Author, 1983.
28. Robert Forman Ph.D., *How to Control Your Allergies* (Larchmont Books, 1979).
29. John Ott, *Light Radiation and You* (Devin Adair, 1982).
30. Kenneth Cooper, *The New Aerobics* (Bantam, 1977).
31. Leon Chaitow, *Your Complete Stress-Proofing Programme* (Thorsons, 1984).
32. Editorial *New England Journal of Medicine*, 10 Dec. 1981; Editorial, *Lancet* 12 Dec. 1981.
33. Dr J. Sorenson 'Therapeutic and Medicinal Uses of Copper Aspirinate', in *Copper: Its Medicinal and Biological Effects* (Academic Press, 1979).
34. Personal Communication to author, 1984.
35. *Journal of Orthomolecular Psychiatry* Vol. 13, No. 2 (1984), pp. 66-93.
36. Betsy Russel Manning, 'How Safe are Mercury Fillings?', Cancer Control Society, Los Angeles, 1984.
37. *Health Consciousness*, April 1984, pp.18-24.
38. *Holistic Medicine* (USA), June-July 1984, p. 29
39. Robert A. Da Prato M.D. '*Fatty acid ion exchange complexes in treatment of Candida Albicans*'. Report by Arteria Co., Concord, California.
40. I. Neuhauser, *Arch. Int. Med* 93: 53-60.

INDEX